ANYBODY CAN DO IT

●

ACUPRESSURE

Leon A. Hart

LYNN MARK
LIBRARY

Library of Congress Catalog Card Number: 76-16924

ISBN 0-918322-01-4

We wish to express our thanks to Mr. Jack Jacoby for his kind help in acquiring reproductions of the Chinese acupuncture sketches.

Published by:

LYNN MARK Library
279 East 44th St.
New York, N.Y. 10017

Printed in the United States of America

First Edition—1977

CONTENTS

SECTION I

HART ACUPRESSURE METHOD

HART ACUPRESSURE METHOD

THE PURPOSE

The purpose of our method is relaxation and concurrent reestablishment of balanced vital energy flow (which means balanced functioning) in the human system. Thus, this book, A*BCDI (Any*Body Can Do It) Acupressure, is built around the simultaneous occurrence of vital energy balance and relaxation—the fact that acupressure massage of vital energy points brings this about, and results in optimum performance of each individual's human system.

All action, mental and physical, is accomplished by means of muscular contraction. It is normal for a living organism to return to repose between contractions (tensions)—as an infant's system does. But due to the stresses of modern life, most adults have lost the capacity to revert to repose, having become slaves of their own tensions. Consequently, they expend vast quantities of energy in nonproductive excessive/unnecessary/chronic tensions. These are the tensions we want to be rid of. And by means of our acupressure relaxation process, we coax the human system back to where it returns to a state of repose between contractions (tensions), thereby eliminating excessive/unnecessary/chronic tensions.

We think of tension as a muscular manifestation, and indeed, tension cannot take place unless muscular contraction occurs. But tension is also a vital energy manifestation and is inevitably accompanied by a disturbance in vital energy balance. When we restore vital energy balance, we automatically restore muscular relaxation. The method

1

whereby we restore this balance is acupressure massage of vital energy points.

But you needn't be concerned with the mechanics in order to benefit from acupressure, you need acknowledge only one precept, which is: **acupressure massage of body points brings about extensive relaxation.** The truth of this statement will become immediately and abundantly obvious to you when you begin applying acupressure.

We must clarify our use of the term "relaxation" in this text—we use the word in its clinical sense, namely: a relaxed muscle is one that's free of all voluntary contractions. (Voluntary refers to those contractions which are subject to control by volition, as opposed to contractions which take place autonomically such as the heartbeat, the propulsion of food through the intestine, and so forth.)

The word "relaxation" is used quite casually in many contexts during everyday conversation—taking a Sunday drive in the country is relaxation from work in an office; watching television is relaxation from working as a truck driver, etc. Such changes of activity are relaxing to some extent but the Sunday driver's brain must still concentrate on driving (which requires muscular contraction) while numerous muscles throughout his body are not only being used but are keyed up (tensed) in readiness for a potential instant response requirement should there be a threatened accident. Watching television requires substantially less active utilization of the musculature, but being slumped in an easy chair in front of a TV does not necessarily mean that the musculature is relaxed—enormous quantities of chronic/excessive tension can be maintained while gazing at the tube. We shall not use relaxation in any casual sense of the term—we will use it only to mean that the musculature is quite free of voluntary contraction.

Tension equals contraction (use), relaxation equals absence of contraction (non-use).

A person functions at his best when the musculature commences an action (contraction) or series of actions from a state of repose (relaxation). The overall objective is to get your system functioning at your top performance level of perfection, and this is done by eliminating interference of (1) tensions (unnecessary/chronic) which are not required in order to accomplish the task at hand, and (2) tensions generated by excessive anxiety about the task.

Tension is the GREAT INTERFERER. Chronically contracted muscles mean only limited function is possible—either much more extreme contraction must take place in order to perform an action, or only a small percentage of the muscle is used to accomplish the action because the rest is too severely knotted.

Even extreme chronic tension does not mean the body will be totally unable to function—it can still perform the necessary actions in the process of living: a head can still be made to turn on a tightly tensed neck, a hand can still hold a pencil and write, legs can still walk. But the functioning will be far below the optimum possible for that individual, will indeed sometimes be downright clumsy.

Let us cite an example: a person's arm and shoulder can be fraught with strong chronic tensions and still perform its routine motions. To demonstrate this to yourself, lift a moderately heavy book (like a dictionary) with your right hand. Note the muscular contractions starting with the hand, through the arm and into the shoulder. Now put the book down, but release the contractions only enough so that you can use your arm and hand. You'll find you can retain an extraordinary number of contractions and still function. Thus you see that the human system can harbor extreme chronic tensions and still manage to perform the basic functions necessary in order to live.

The problem is that it's a needless strain on the musculature to have to form its contractions around, above, and in spite of the chronic contractions already present. But more importantly, although the muscles still manage to accomplish elementary functions, in any situation where they may be expected to perform with optimum efficiency —such as in sports competition—they're going to be severely hampered by the chronic contractions, and won't give anywhere near the kind of performance they'd be capable of if they started from a state of repose. Indeed, sports is one of the areas in which you'll note startling improvement in your abilities after you've succeeded in releasing some of your tensions. In ice hockey, for instance, chronic underlying tensions make precision response of the

3

musculature impossible, thus undermining your game. Or let that severely contracted arm and shoulder in which there's still sufficient mobility to do everyday things like combing hair or eating food be required to perform in a tennis match. Then the extent to which those chronic contractions interfere will become very obvious.

Not only tensions of physical origin but also those of mental origin will interfere with peak performance. You know that when you're laden with mental/emotional anxieties, it's difficult to concentrate on something which requires full attention. Mental anxiety/tension interferes with both optimum mental and physical performance, just as physical tension does. Therefore, the alleviation of mental anxiety is as vital toward achieving top performance as is relief of physical tension. Acupressure relaxation of the musculature is the least expensive and easiest way to relieve mental anxiety. In order for anxiety to take place, muscular contraction (tension) must take place—if the required contractions are not present, the anxiety does not occur. Relaxation, combined with removal of oneself from the cause of the problem, provides the most expeditious means of anxiety relief.

In acupressure, we have an extraordinarily potent means of relaxing excessive/unnecessary/chronic tensions of both mental and physical origin. By resolving these tensions, we not only eliminate interference, we also put a stop to the waste of enormous quantities of vital energy. These large amounts of energy are required to maintain excessive/chronic tensions. By stopping the waste, your full store of energy becomes available for productive use. Thus, your powerhouse of vital energy is under your own control by means of simple massage manipulation of your acupoints.

When you function from a base of relaxation, there is an appropriateness of energy in all your actions—everything you do is accomplished by using only the required amount of energy, but using that amount fully, to its ultimate capacity, so as to achieve peak performance. Relaxation permits the body systems to function at their normal momentum to their optimum potential.

By practicing the acupressure techniques, one learns to

4

relax completely and at will. Our purpose is to return the human system to that natural condition where it is able to revert to repose between tensions (actions)—as an infant's system does. Acupressure massage of vital energy points is utilized by acupuncture therapists in treatment of illness, but this is not the intent of our text. We do not have medical aims for the direct cure or alleviation of any disease conditions with the Hart method. Relaxation, of and by itself, does, of course, aid in the alleviation or cure of numerous physical and mental ailments, but any sort of direct treatment of illness is beyond the realm of this book.

Our intent is the following: to explain a simple pressure-massage technique which is extraordinarily effective in relieving tensions. We wish to provide the human being with this uncomplicated, completely safe, yet startlingly powerful means of relaxation, in order to help people achieve, as nearly as possible, total relaxation—or zero repose. Our purpose is to provide these techniques for normal persons who wish to improve, through relaxation, their ability to handle the inevitable stresses of living. Massage manipulation of vital energy points is the method by which we achieve relaxation, since relaxation and vital energy balance occur simultaneously. And when the body regains its ability to relax (return to balance) between contractions, this results in optimum performance of each individual's human system.

Therefore, by way of acupressure, the Hart Method provides a means not only for dealing with stress/tension/anxiety, but also for achieving one's ultimate performance capability and for attaining the fullest participation in the life experience. And this is, in the final analysis, what we all want—to work and function at the peak of our capacity and to enjoy the fullest possible experience of living. Tension is the Great Interferer. Unnecessary/excessive/chronic tensions interfere in multitudinous ways with our ability to function fully. Acupressure relaxation techniques are our means of combatting the insidious takeover of our systems by such tensions. Thereby we are able to eliminate interference and return to our natural capacity for optimum achievement and total participation in life.

5

SOME BENEFITS OF ACUPRESSURE RELAXATION

Following is a list of some specific ways in which acupressure relaxation can help you. In truth, the number of ways is almost unlimited and you'll observe all kinds of benefits, including many which we haven't listed, in your own individual situation.

1. Earn More Money
2. Look Younger
3. Learn to Know Yourself
4. Learn to Know Others
5. Achieve Harmonious Living (In Accord With Your Biorhythm)
6. Fulfill Your Optimum Potential
7. Achieve Total Creative Expression
8. Make the Most Efficient and Productive Use of Your Energy
9. Improve Your Performance
10. Improve Your Learning Capabilities
11. Improve Your Memory
12. Achieve Remarkable New Mental Acuity
13. Achieve Mental Serenity
14. Enjoy Increased Sensory Response
15. Rid Yourself of Nervous Tension, Anxiety, Fearfulness
16. Reduce Irritability
17. Improve Your Understanding and Acceptance of Life
18. Achieve Resilience Against Stress/Pressure
19. Tension-Caused Aches and Pains Will Vanish

20. **Prevent Excessive Nervous Perspiration**
21. **Enjoy Optimum Digestive Function**
22. **Posture Will Improve**
23. **You'll Breathe Properly**
24. **Sleep Better**
25. **Acupressure Reestablishes Balanced Functioning of Autonomic Systems**

Let's expand briefly on each of the foregoing.

1. EARN MORE MONEY. Although "the best things in life are free", things like food and shelter cost money. In our modern society, the standard of life we enjoy depends on our ability to pay. If we earn more, we can pay more. Acupressure relaxation helps you earn more.

Tension can, and usually does, interfere with every aspect of your work performance. It impedes intellectual function, disrupts muscle coordination, and, as an inevitable result, undermines self-confidence. Removal of tension interference brings improvement in everything you do, so you perform better at your present job, and are able to undertake more demanding tasks and responsibility at higher salary in advanced positions.

For example:

If you are an executive—you'll find decision-making easier and more forceful after you've rid yourself of excessive/chronic tensions. When muscles are knotted with chronic contractions, they cannot fully perform the contractions necessary for total utilization of brain power in decision-making. Muscle contraction is required in order for any mental process to take place and chronic underlying contractions interfere with mental ability to perform just as they interfere with physical ability to perform.

As you achieve relaxation, you'll experience expanded intellectual capacity to grasp new material. Being able to absorb information quickly and make decisions efficiently will increase your self-confidence. As all aspects of your work improve, you'll gain total belief in yourself. And when you believe in yourself, you've got the greatest power on Earth working for you.

If you are a pianist—you'll find yourself playing with surprising new facility as you gain relaxation. You'll be memorizing material more rapidly—your interpretations will be fuller, richer, and have greater insight. (The same holds true if you are any other type of musician.) When you play better, your earning potential is increased.

If you are a secretary—typing ease and speed will increase as you remove interfering tensions. Your all-around memory, concentration, and competence will improve, giving you a feeling of remarkable new confidence which will encourage you to seek more responsibility at greater pay.

Regardless of what your occupation may be, excessive/unnecessary/chronic tension is your Great Interferer. Remove those tensions and your capacities can function at their fullest—which means raises, promotions, and better jobs will come your way.

2. **LOOK YOUNGER.** Tension frequently causes people to look many years older than they need to. Chronic contractions pulling the face into fixed anxiety-ridden expressions will undeniably cause a person to look older than when his face is serene and relaxed. Age occurs eventually and is inevitable, but when tension plays havoc with a person's face, the look of age occurs much sooner than necessary. Through simple relaxation, a young, smooth, serene visage can be maintained well on into the late years of life.

3. **LEARN TO KNOW YOURSELF.** When you are relaxed, you are at one with yourself—excessive/chronic tensions and anxieties constitute a barrier between you and yourself, making it difficult or impossible for you to communicate with yourself. Tension causes you to live at odds with yourself. You are forced to carry on a running battle with your own tensions.

Relaxation removes the barrier. You and yourself are suddenly face to face with each other, revealing all the elements of your being, right down to the minutest detail. It is a marvellous revelation—learning to know yourself. And it is a source of infinite strength—from the very inception of Earth's greatest civilizations, the wise have said "know yourself". For they recognized the power a human attains through self-knowledge.

4. LEARN TO KNOW OTHERS. When you are relaxed and free of anxiety/tension-caused conflicts, your ability to analyze, assess, and deal with others is vastly increased. You become able to see the conflicts others are suffering, you recognize their ambitions and schemes, you see where you can influence a situation and when it is worthwhile to do so. At the same time, you recognize those situations where it is not worth your time and effort to deal with them, and consequently, that they should be circumvented or ignored.

Your capacity for handling people is enhanced since, when you operate from a base of relaxation, you're much calmer in your approach, more serene in your attitudes. You'll find yourself stronger, more in command of any situation that may arise.

5. ACHIEVE HARMONIOUS LIVING (IN ACCORD WITH YOUR BIORHYTHM). Relaxation establishes balance; balance is harmony. Through relaxation, you improve and preserve your physical and mental health —because an organism which functions in balance according to its natural rhythm (in harmony) avoids and/or removes the myriad ailments which tension engenders.

Relaxation promotes a harmonious life-style in rhythm with both your inner self and your external environment.

6. FULFILL YOUR OPTIMUM POTENTIAL. When you're at one with yourself, free of internal conflicts, you'll suddenly be operating at full capacity. This is inevitably a fantastically gratifying experience. When you've learned how to do away with the excessive/unnecessary/chronic tensions which cause conflicts and blockages to exist, when you know how to avoid future development of such tensions, you'll come to this startling realization of your own potential. The outcome will be a new, serene self-assurance, as you calmly, unhurriedly, proceed to fulfill that potential.

7. ACHIEVE TOTAL CREATIVE EXPRESSION.

Tension is THE Great Interferer in the realm of creativity. Its interference here is perhaps more devastating and problematic than in any other area of human endeavor. You can drive a bus, cook a meal, preside over a board meeting, dispatch trucks, you can perform just about all the motions of living while maintaining severe chronic tensions throughout your body. But your creative talents will be shot—or hampered to the point where they might as well be shot. Tension impedes or prevents the expression of creativity.

If tension has been blocking your creative powers, the release will be like a burst of light. In order for creativity to work, the subconscious must be employed. Tension effectively stymies feedback between the conscious and subconscious. The removal of tension opens the lines of communication, making total creative expression a reality.

8. MAKE THE MOST EFFICIENT AND PRODUCTIVE USE OF YOUR ENERGY.

Actions performed from a state of repose (relaxation) utilize only as much as, not more than, the energy required to accomplish a specific action. Thus energy conservation is achieved. Using only that amount of energy (tension) required for each task means the most efficient use of your resources, avoidance of wasted energy, and prevention of needless wear and tear on your human system. As a result, you'll feel like you've just had a great new injection of energy into your system.

9. IMPROVE YOUR PERFORMANCE.

This has already been mentioned since it occurs as part of numerous benefits, but it's so vital of and by itself that it should be emphasized by giving it separate status. When tension no longer interferes, overall operation of your entire human system improves. You'll find yourself doing better at all the skill-requiring things you've done for years—whether it be writing plays, singing country music, target shooting, swimming, carpentry, driving an automobile, programming a computer, or whatever. Simple acupressure relaxation brings about this remarkable, highly visible betterment in performance.

11

10. IMPROVE YOUR LEARNING CAPABILITIES.

Although of particular importance to students, all of us must keep on learning throughout our adult years if we want to get ahead in life. Therefore, superior learning ability is exceedingly valuable to just about everyone. But if you are presently a student, your immediate concern is, of course, the matter of finishing school with the best possible grade average. Tension/anxiety gets credit for the greatest interference in the learning process. Simple removal of that tension eliminates the roadblocks, leaving the way clear for top-level effectuation of your mental capabilities. Consequently, you're free to achieve that best possible grade average.

Your ability to learn better and more easily will persist throughout life as long as you continue to monitor your system in order to avoid takeover by chronic/unnecessary/ excessive tensions. When you notice such tensions creeping in, they must be ousted by practicing relaxation techniques.

11. IMPROVE YOUR MEMORY.

Tension interferes with recall. Your information storage depot is your subconscious, and tension impedes communication between your conscious and subconscious.

We might illustrate by use of a simple, rather common example: when you're trying to remember a word or somebody's name and you strain in trying, it usually doesn't come. Later, when the effort has been relaxed and your mind is loose, the name or word quickly comes.

12. ACHIEVE REMARKABLE NEW MENTAL ACUITY.

Excessive/unnecessary/chronic tensions undermine the mental processes. Relaxation restores full and proper function.

Upon removal of tension interference, your mental awareness will improve and you'll enjoy greater alertness with increased powers of perception and concentration. You'll find your ability to think and reason remarkably enhanced. The mind will work more smoothly and efficiently, with a minimum of effort (meaning only the truly necessary energy expenditure will take place). And due to your new mental ease, your brain will experience fresh flexibility which enables it to find innovative solutions to difficult problems.

13. ACHIEVE MENTAL SERENITY. Relaxation engenders a gratifying mental serenity due in large part to the tranquil confidence that one can cope with any problems which may arise. Thereupon follows a more optimistic and cheerful outlook on life.

14. ENJOY INCREASED SENSORY RESPONSE. Tension inhibits sensory response. Upon elimination of tension interference, the sensory apparatus is free to function totally—which means you see, hear, smell better.

15. RID YOURSELF OF NERVOUS TENSION, ANXIETY, FEARFULNESS. It is impossible to be anxious, fearful, upset, when you are relaxed. Muscular contraction (tension) is required in order for anxiety/fear-laden mental states to take place. If you relax the tension, the emotional state ceases to exist. If this seems incredible, you need only try it to prove it to yourself. Relax yourself completely. Then try worrying anxiously about something—you can feel yourself having to tense muscles in order to worry.

Thus relaxation brings about direct reduction of anxiety. This results in reduced compulsion to worry needlessly, and engenders a feeling of self-sufficiency and independence. Inordinate anxiety tends to make one feel inadequate, unable to cope, and is conducive toward heavy leaning on others.

16. REDUCE IRRITABILITY. Excessive chronic anxiety/tension usually makes a person irritable and prone to emotional outbursts. The next time you have to deal with someone who's given to temper tantrums, observe his behavior between outbursts. You'll probably see without difficulty the tensions coursing through him, and their volatility as they explode in fits of irritation or temper. Regular practice of relaxation techniques can relieve the causative anxiety.

17. IMPROVE YOUR UNDERSTANDING AND ACCEPTANCE OF LIFE. Relaxation will bring a better comprehension and acceptance of the conditions of life. Out of this will evolve a calmer "philosophical" approach toward those afflictions and misfortunes over which a person has no control.

18. **ACHIEVE RESILIENCE AGAINST STRESS/PRESSURE.** Each human being has an inborn capacity for withstanding impressively large quantities of stress. When basically relaxed and in balance, the human system can undergo periods of super-intense stress (tension) without ill effect. It is this natural resilience which relaxation permits you to regain.

19. **TENSION-CAUSED ACHES AND PAINS WILL VANISH.** Tension is a frequent cause of aches throughout the human body, headache being, no doubt, the most common of such pains.

Where the cause is tension, the cure is relaxation.

20. **PREVENT EXCESSIVE NERVOUS PERSPIRATION.** Continuous nervous tension ordinarily results in perennially clammy palms and perspiration-wet feet. While a tense person is sleeping, it also causes excessive perspiration of the back from the neck to the waist, to the point where the pillow case and bottom sheet are wet in the morning. Since nervous tension is the cause of the problem, relaxation is the solution.

21. **ENJOY OPTIMUM DIGESTIVE FUNCTION.** It's well known that tense, hostile arguments at the dinner table will adversely affect the digestive process. By the same token, chronic tensions often cause chronic digestive problems. In order to function at optimum efficiency, the digestive system must be free and relaxed.

22. **POSTURE WILL IMPROVE.** The depression/frustration which often accompanies anxiety/tension will usually result in stooped, dejected posture. On the other hand, a relaxed body will function with natural excellence of bearing, automatically balanced on its center of gravity. This lends great vitality, besides giving the body a more youthful look.

23. **YOU'LL BREATHE PROPERLY.** Relaxation means proper breathing. A tense body cannot breathe fully; a relaxed body cannot do anything but breathe fully.

When tense, breathing is shallow, short, uneven—using

only a small portion of lung capacity. When relaxed, the lungs are free to operate fully. You don't need to learn how to breathe, your lungs know how. All you need do is relax them so they are completely free to function without interference. In fact, in order to make your lungs breathe improperly, you must interfere by tensing up. If your lungs are tension-free and loose, they automatically breathe correctly.

24. **SLEEP BETTER.** When you've accomplished basic relaxation, you'll sleep better and your body will renew itself more efficiently while you are sleeping. Consequently, you'll feel stronger, more energetic during waking hours.

However, it should be borne in mind that relaxation does not, cannot, and will not take the place of sleep. There are proponents of certain relaxation methods who state that if you practice their method, one of your benefits will be that you'll require less sleep (therefore you'll be able to do either more work or more partying, depending upon your inclination). The contention is that a few minutes of said relaxation will revitalize your system as would a full night's sleep. This is not possible. The purpose of sleep is to permit the body time to do its repair work. It cannot do in twenty minutes what it has been genetically programmed to do in approximately seven hours (for most people), no matter how completely you relax during those twenty minutes. Consequently, don't expect a relaxation session, regardless of the method you use, to take the place of your normal sleep requirement.

As your whole system becomes more relaxed, you may find that you sleep an hour or two less than formerly, but the vast majority of people will find that they sleep longer than they did prior to practicing relaxation. Which will happen depends on what your natural requirements are, and on how severely, and in what direction, tension had been interfering with your natural needs. Most people find they sleep more when relaxed because many more people are kept awake by tension than are inclined to sleep excessively due to tension. Pharmaceutical firms sell a far greater quantity of drugs for putting people to sleep than

15

for keeping people awake. The greater problem is insomnia, not excessive sleep. And the major cause of insomnia is anxiety/tension.

There are some individuals who sleep incredibly well in spite of extreme tension throughout their bodies. These persons find in sleep an escape from life; often the only thing they really enjoy doing is sleeping. Such individuals will inevitably sleep less when their anxiety/tensions have been relieved.

A healthy, relaxed body automatically sleeps the proper number of hours required for body-rebuilding, the length of time varying in accordance with each person's inherent needs. When relaxed, the human system can reap the utmost benefit out of sleep, thus natural rhythm is restored as normal sleep requirement is met. Excellent sleep, in the proper amount, gives rise to a wonderful feeling of well-being as you enjoy the blessings of a rested body and mind.

25. **REESTABLISH BALANCED FUNCTIONING OF AUTONOMIC SYSTEMS.** Tension/anxiety throws autonomic systems off-balance; relaxation reestablishes their natural balanced functioning. These systems control automatic motor functions of the body, such as digestion, circulation and so forth. (In essence, all functions of the body which occur automatically without your conscious volition are autonomic.)

The removal of excessive/unnecessary/chronic tension, and the balanced autonomic function which comes as a result thereof, can help avert what are perhaps the two most common physical ailments brought on by psychic tension/anxiety: ulcer (stomach, intestinal) and cardiovascular disease (hypertension, heartattack). The effect of tension (stress) on cardiovascular and gastrointestinal function is well known—the benefit of relaxation is undeniable.

ACUPRESSURE

DEVELOPMENT OF THE METHOD

Since his beginning, the human being has instinctively used his hands to massage his tense sore muscles. I, being human, have done exactly that. And out of this natural action grew the following method of acupressure massage.

In the process of developing this method, my experience was that overall human tension, both physical and psychic, manifests itself strongly in the face—in facial muscles generally and more acutely in small spots or points within the muscles. By massaging these tension areas and points in the face, one could effectively relieve physical tension throughout the entire body, as well as psychic tension.

The method later became expanded to include massage of areas and points on the neck, shoulders, arms and legs. In every instance, it was observed that relaxation was not confined solely to the small area of massage, but spread itself throughout the entire human system.

Thus it became clear that total mental/physical tension could be relieved by a simple method of massage which concentrates action, particularly pressure, on small specific areas and points.

The inseparable interdependence of mind and body also became abundantly clear through observation of the manner in which both mental and physical tensions relaxed simultaneously as a result of massage applied to those areas and points.

This absolute intertwining of the total human organism caused me to search for a term expressing mind/body together as an entity. The two are so efficiently separated in Western thinking, we don't even have a word which may be used to denote them together as one Whole. It therefore became advisable to assign some term to signify body/mind as a total inseparable unit. The term "human system" seemed a simple solution. It's true that "system" is sometimes used to denote the physical body as a functioning mechanism, but this usage is not so ingrained that it precludes using "human system" to denote body and mind as one inseparable unit. Therefore, when we use the term "human system" in this book we refer to human mind/body as a complete Whole—indivisible, it being impossible to influence one without also influencing the other.

With regard to the term "acupressure"—I began using this word rather recently as a result of acupuncture research and the realization that the pressure points I was using were vital energy (acupuncture) points. Previously, I'd simply call the method "pressure massage", a name derived from the important role pressure played in most all manipulations employed.

While developing this acupressure method, I found myself using the various massage techniques of pressing, rubbing, pinching, squeezing, and hammering (percussion). Most Americans have had little or no experience with professional massage; usually it's been limited to having had a friend or relative rub the back of a tense neck. Mine, too, had been limited to just that. Nevertheless, when developing massage techniques, I intuitively used the same manipulatory motions employed by professional masseurs in modern as well as ancient massage methods. There is nothing impressive in this—massage techniques are instinctive to the human being, and basically the same techniques are used in the various professional, as well as nonprofessional, methods. Ancient massage methods practiced by widely separated civilizations were likewise essentially similar to each other, and are similar to modern systems.

My primary reason for the preceding paragraph is to impress you with the validity of your own instincts. Because massage is such a simple process of rubbing, squeezing, pressing, and tapping, we're inclined to think "it's so simple, how can it do any good?". But it does do good—an enormous amount of good. People who've had little contact with massage often have the feeling there must be some special secret, some mysterious something that only the "masters" can do, and the massage they themselves do could not possibly be of much benefit. Not so. It's true a professional may have a certain procedure for approaching specific pathological muscle-tension problems, and, if trained in the areas involved, would know how to alleviate certain medical problems. But we are concerned in this book with normally healthy people having only the usual everyday tensions, and such a person can do himself a vast amount of good by simply following his instincts and the suggestions put forth in this book. That plain, ordinary rubbing, squeezing and pressing which you do can be enormously beneficial to you. Your intuition encourages you to do massage. Believe in your intuition.

The enlightened wisdom of ancient civilizations considered massage to be the most natural or instinctual of restorative techniques. We must learn to recognize anew the remarkable therapeutic value of simple massage.

In addition to its innate simplicity, there's another facet of this therapy we should discuss—that is the fact that most of us are inclined to think of massage as something someone else does to us. Of course, it is often done by one person to another, especially today, when people incline toward believing a person must be a "specialist" to perform massage. But "specialization" is not really necessary in order to press, rub, squeeze, and tap the skin of the body. Anybody can do it. You can do it on your own tension spots, and it's extraordinarily effective in promoting relaxation.

We certainly admit there are limitations to how extensive a traditional Western-style massage you could give yourself since, in this method, entire large-muscle areas are manipulated by one motion, areas such as the full-muscle of the calf, or of the forearm. But as you perform massage, you'll soon see that full-muscle manipulation by a single massage action is not really necessary—massaging parts of the muscle area, one part at a time, effectively and efficiently relaxes the entire muscle, plus the rest of the musculature of your entire body. And as you proceed to develop that small-area manipulation into the even more defined action of vital energy point massage, you'll find the relaxation effect in the individual muscle area enormously increased, with a corresponding, simultaneous increase in relaxation throughout your entire system.

Vital energy point massage, like Western massage, is often performed by one person on another. But we are convinced that when you perform acupressure on yourself, you gain a tremendous advantage over having someone else massage you. When doing it yourself you're able to utilize the fact that you can sense exactly how your muscles are reacting at all times—you know how much pressure to apply, you feel when you've done enough, you can monitor your reactions on a continuing basis. If someone else massages you, that person has to judge how much to massage a particular area, or ask how the area feels when manipulated and try to gauge by what is said. Of course, a professional masseur can tell by touch when a muscle is knotted or badly tensed, but the advantages of doing your own massage go far beyond that. You always feel how each muscle or body point is responding, you feel how sore (tense) it might be, you feel just how much rubbing, squeezing, pressing or tapping a particular muscular area or point can take before it should be left alone for a while so it has time to adjust to its new relaxation and recuperate from suddenly finding itself flexible after being so long in a state of chronic tension.

An objection to doing your own acupressure might be that you can't reach many areas on your back. This is true, but the back is the only part beyond your reach and it is, in fact, not really necessary to massage points there. Only a few key points or areas of the body need be treated in order to achieve excellent general relaxation. While developing this acupressure method, I intuitively excluded all areas on the trunk, in front as well as in back. Using areas and points on the head, shoulders, neck, arms and legs provides effective overall relaxation of the entire human system. It never seemed necessary or even advisable to massage body points on the trunk itself. Doing points on the face, neck and appendages seemed to be the desirable means of eliminating tension in the many organs and organ systems located in the trunk because of an obvious sphere of influence throughout the human system for each body point massaged. The preferred approach presented itself as treatment of points removed from the trunk but involving the trunk in their spheres of influence. The observation was that every point on head, neck, arms, and legs has extensive influence—first, an overall influence throughout the human system, and secondly, a stronger, specific sphere of influence involving a specific body area or organ system.

When first developing this acupressure method, I was quite intrigued by the manner in which massage on one minute point invariably exerted a potent influence over a large part of the human system. Massage on points around the mouth, for example, has a powerful sphere of influence right down the center of the torso, being especially strong in the reproductive organs.

Recently, with the sudden dissemination of knowledge about acupuncture into the United States, I learned why manipulation of small spots or points on the skin, particularly applying pressure to these points, has such an extensive sphere of influence. The small spots are the vital energy points used in acupuncture, and the spheres of influence are due to vital energy circulation throughout the body and predominantly along meridians.

Until former President Nixon's trip to Peking in 1972, I, along with millions of other Americans, had never heard of acupuncture or vital energy points. I had no idea there was any such therapeutic system. Upon first reading about acupuncture in newspapers, I immediately accepted it as valid because the mind said—"those are the same body points I've been using in pressure massage". Later, when doing research on acupuncture, I was nevertheless surprised to discover the extent of the similarities between it and what I'd devised as a massage system. Not that a system of gaining benefit by massaging or otherwise manipulating specific points on the body is so difficult to come

21

upon—over the past 6,000 years-plus of human history, many persons, independently of one another, have hit upon therapy methods which involved use of body points and meridians. How humanity utilized these methods, or failed to utilize them, was dependent on three factors: 1) the circumstances under which a particular method was discovered, 2) the intelligence and education of the discoverer, and 3) the particular problem alleviated or cured at the time of the discovery. Some examples of independently-discovered uses of body points in medical diagnosis and therapy are mentioned in the section on acupuncture. But despite the fact that various means of body point utilization have been hit upon at different times throughout history and my discovery was not entirely unique, it was still a pleasant surprise to have the effectiveness of my homely massage method corroborated by the ancient, venerable system of acupuncture therapy.

The express purpose in describing the way my acupressure method developed intuitively many years before I knew anything about acupuncture with its body points and vital energy is to make clear that these massage techniques and their effects are natural impulses. The method grew out of natural actions and reactions, it was not devised in limbo somewhere and then imposed on the human system. The method is an expansion and formalization of what is, in fact, intuitive knowledge—it was not contrived extrinsic to innate human behavior. Acupressure massage, then, as well as acupuncture therapy are the result of a reality which exists within the human system. They are means of influencing that reality of body points and vital energy circulation.

In this book, we will first present the complete method of acupressure as it was created for personal use. Then, in the following section, we will talk about acupuncture therapy and its relation to body point massage.

VITAL ENERGY POINTS

DISCOVERY OF THE POINTS

I felt a good deal of tension focusing itself in my face, especially in the eyebrows (I was inclined to frown in fervent concentration) and around the mouth (I was inclined to maintain a stiff upper lip while frowning in fervent concentration). I began rubbing and applying pressure to the face to relieve some of this tightness and discovered the small, specific spots where it felt particularly beneficial to apply pressure. I pressed these spots with fingers and knuckles. It seemed the benefit would be increased if pressure were better centralized and so I sought an implement of narrow diameter to use. The handle of an artist's paint brush turned out to be a fine implement and pressure applied with it was indeed more beneficial.

I found similar spots on the neck and shoulders which responded admirably to pressure massage. Pressing and rubbing tight muscles in the legs also revealed such spots there. Combining the various massage techniques of rubbing, pinching, and pressing, concentrated on and around these sites, proved extraordinarily conducive to achieving relaxation. This was the manner in which I discovered the minute spots on the body which are known as vital energy points.

Later, on examining some ancient acupuncture charts, it was interesting indeed to see many of these points noted. All are not noted since acupuncture charts usually indicate only the points on the 14 major meridians, which comes to but a small fraction of the total points on the body.

When you rub or press tense muscles, the sensation you feel is soreness. When you rub or press a tension-sensitized vital energy point, you feel a slightly different kind of soreness—like a focalization of the soreness. It was this unique focalized sensation at the points which made it possible to discover their precise locations—although an

23

entire muscular area felt sore when tense, the soreness centralized itself in these very specific, small points.

To clarify the type of soreness to which we refer: when a muscle area anywhere on the body is sore with tension, it'll feel the way the muscles in the back of the neck, right at the shoulders, feel when tense. We use this example because virtually everyone has rubbed or massaged the back of his neck when it was tense, or had someone rub it for him, and knows from that experience how tension-sore muscles feel. This sensation is different from the soreness of a sprained ankle, burnt finger, etc. It is the soreness resulting from tension with which we're concerned in this book, not the kind of soreness associated with burns, sprains, bruises, infections, or any other such thing.

If you massage a vital energy point in which tension is centralized anywhere on the body, you'll feel tension-soreness. If there is no tension related to a particular point, tension-soreness will not be present.

With further experience, I discovered that there are several body points where "point sensation" is present even when there is no tension in the muscle or point and consequently no soreness of muscle or point. The feeling of point sensation is entirely different from that of point tension-soreness. How a relaxed body point which possesses point sensation feels when pressed may be analogously described as follows: if you take an area of skin where your muscles are relaxed and squeeze it between your thumb and forefinger, you will feel a sensation which will not be soreness (unless you squeeze too hard, in which case you'll get pain and a bruise, so squeeze gently). But if you take an area of skin where your muscles are tense and tight and squeeze it between your thumb and forefinger, it will feel sore. In a like manner, pressure on relaxed body points—those where sensation is always present—will produce point sensation but no soreness. However, if a point has been sensitized by tension, it will feel sore when pressure is applied just as tense muscles feel sore.

The fact that many body points can be felt (have point

sensation) when pressed even though the person is relaxed and healthy, is normal.

Illness produces several other reactions at body points. In some cases, certain points will become spontaneously painful. In other cases, depending on the ailment, specific points may become inflamed, lumpy, hot, cold, raised, painful on light or average pressure, or otherwise pathologically influenced. Any such conditions at body points may indicate malfunction of some organ or system. If there is spontaneous overt discomfort at a body point, or any pain, don't massage that point.

In all illnesses, whether of a physical or mental nature, there will be certain vital energy points on the skin which present various symptoms, including any of the abovementioned. When the illness is cured, symptoms at the body points will vanish. Acupuncture therapy is one means of curing numerous ailments and thereby removing symptoms at points. However, symptoms will disappear regardless of how the cure was achieved; whether the human system simply healed itself in time, or whether drugs, herbs, suggestion, or any other therapeutic method was used to aid in healing.

When illness and/or tension are no longer present, the body points will either have no sensation at all when pressed (nor any pathological symptoms) or they will have only normal point sensation (if they are among those points which usually have such sensation).

To summarize, the various conditions possible at body points are as follows:

1. No sensation at all. In this case you will, of course, not be able to find the point without having had special training.
2. Point sensation. These are the spots where the point sensation described above is always present. This is normal for these points.
3. Soreness which is present as a result of simple tension. This is essentially the same type of soreness as is present in your muscles as a result of simple tension—the soreness focalizes itself in the points.

25

4. Symptoms such as inflammation, pain, etc, which may indicate a pathological malfunction.

It is condition #3 with which we're concerned in our acupressure massage method. It's our aim to do away with the anxiety/tension which causes this soreness.

The ideal body condition is one where vital energy points either produce no sensation when pressed, or produce only point sensation and no other symptoms are present. Under the normal stresses of living, however, it's questionable whether this ideal state is often achieved—most of us don't choose to lead a static life in which we never participate in adventure or risk. And most of us don't have the financial resources to lead a static life even if we chose to do so—we're obliged to earn a living and doing this inevitably involves some stress. Body points will reflect the conditions of our lives.

It is not our intention to do away with stress, our aim is simply to help the human system return to relaxation between stresses. It's our opinion that stress is a normal and desirable ingredient of life, that a static existence is not what God had in mind for the human being. But stress must be tempered by periods of repose. The human system should return to zero repose, or close to it, between its stressful involvements.

Infants and animals automatically revert to repose between stresses, but due to the nature of our modern technological existence, most adults have lost this ability. It's because stress/tension/anxiety tends to become the chronic state in today's living environment that people need to learn certain techniques for regaining their ability to return to repose between stress episodes. Of the several relaxation methods available for personal use, acupressure massage applied to vital energy points is far and away the most powerful and effective single method for breaking chronic tension and easing repose.

HOW TO LOCATE POINTS

We've stated that it's acupoint condition #3—soreness at the points resulting from simple tension—with which we're concerned. Finding these points is a relatively simple

26

matter. To begin with, you can sense the general area where you have tension. It may be your forehead. Rub the entire area with your fingers or knuckles. When you feel certain small spots where tension-soreness is centralized, you've located the points. Besides tension-soreness, you may find a slight nodule at the site, or a little strip of tense, hard muscle. If you use acupressure massage at that point directly on the hard strip of muscle, the hardness will eventually disappear as tension is reduced. I recall having had small, hard strips of muscle in some points along the eyebrows. These have since vanished as the brows relaxed.

The size of various points on the body differs substantially—most are minute but some may be as large as 3/16 of an inch in diameter. Those on the face are quite small; whereas on the legs, there are some we use in acupressure which are noticeably larger.

When massaging or locating acupoints, always use gentle pressure, do not use heavy, severe pressure. Tension soreness can be felt by applying mild pressure, don't ever think that you have to press down hard in order to find tension or vital energy points. If you press hard enough anywhere on your body, you're going to get the beginnings of a pain sensation, and if you press so hard as to injure (bruise) yourself, you're definitely going to get pain. Pain is nature's alarm signal that injury is imminent or actually occurring. Pressing hard enough to get pain is not the way to determine locations of acupressure points. You will feel the sensation at the points (if sensation is present) with only limited pressure.

Just as it is true that only gentle pressure is required to locate points, it's also true that only gentle pressure is needed when massaging points. In our acupressure method, all massage actions should be gentle but firm.

POINTS ARE BILATERAL

With the exception of those down the center front or center back of the body, all vital energy points are bilateral (each is located in the same position on both sides of the body). It won't be unusual to find that a point is tension-

27

sore on one side of your body while the corresponding point on the other side is not tense. As is well known, each side of the human system functions to a certain extent independently of the other. There may be substantial tension on one side of the face, for instance, but only little on the opposite side. A common, everyday example of this phenomenon is the fact that tension headaches often affect primarily one side of the head.

It's an interesting experience to feel point soreness on one side of the body and not on the other. To illustrate, at this moment I can feel, by pressing with my index finger, a point behind my right ear, but I cannot feel the same point on the left side. This is obviously one of the points which can't be felt unless tension or some other equilibrium-disturbing factor is present. I'm aware of some general tension on the right side of my head, which is, in this case, the equilibrium-disturbing factor. (On doing the final draft of this book several weeks after writing the above lines, I tried pressing the same area behind the right ear—no point sensation whatever. The tension which had caused point soreness to be present has completely subsided.)

In the course of this text on acupressure, we'll usually refer to a point in the singular but the reference will include its corresponding point on the opposite side of the body. Exceptions might occur when we specifically differentiate by indicating a point on the right or left side, (as in the brief anecdote above) or when the context necessitates referring to both points using the plural.

SPHERES OF INFLUENCE, OR MERIDIANS

As you work with your vital energy points, you'll experience the sphere of influence which reaches substantially beyond a point's own immediate location, in addition to a lesser, generalized influence over your entire system. The sphere of influence is the meridian of acupuncture. Although important traditional meridians incorporate only a small percentage of the total points, each one of the well over a thousand points on the body is connected or related in some way with a sphere of influence. In addition to the fourteen traditional meridians (12 organ plus Conception Vessel and Governor Vessel), there are peripheral and connecting meridians, minor meridians, and non-specific meridians. Acupuncture therapy recognizes the existence of them all, but it's primarily the points on the 14 major ones which most directly influence the organs or organ systems treated in acupuncture. We will find, too, that many of the acupressure body points we use are located on the major meridians.

When applying acupressure on points, any of the following may occur:

1. If there is soreness at a body point, you may either feel sensation along a substantial length of that point's meridian, or you may feel no meridian sensation. (Presence of tension-soreness at the point does not automatically mean meridian sensation will occur.)
2. If there's no soreness but there is point sensation, you may feel slight sensation along some part of the meridian. The foregoing is true for only a very small number of points; usually, if there is only point sensation, you'll feel no sensation along the meridian.
3. If there's no sensation of any kind at the point, you'll feel no sensation along the meridian.

Regardless of whether manipulation of a tension-sore point produces actual sensation along a meridian or not, you will still feel reaction in the form of relaxation taking place in the organs or systems influenced by that point.

Meridians may seem a bit confused at the moment but that's not important since you needn't know them in order to use acupressure. The material is here just for your information, so you can recognize meridian sensation when it occurs. All you need know in using acupressure effectively is 1) that vital energy points exist, 2) the location of a few major points, 3) what massage techniques to employ on the points, and 4) when you apply point massage you will feel relaxation taking place, that you'll have an inclination to relax further throughout substantial areas of the body, and that you should go along fully with this inclination. It's very simple. Anybody can do it.

The reason this acupressure method works is that point massage influences vital energy which is the reflective, formative and controlling force of the human system (yes, all at the same time, although it seems contradictory). By influencing this force, all aspects of human function are influenced—an obvious and direct result being relaxation of the musculature and cerebrospinal-autonomic nervous system.

THE METHOD

As noted earlier, both the inclination to do massage and the techniques involved are intuitive. When developing this acupressure method, I used the same fundamental actions usually employed, namely 1) pressure, 2) movement, 3) friction, and 4) percussion. Since I'd personally never had experience with professional massage and hadn't researched the subject at that time, I didn't know what techniques were utilized—I only did what came naturally, and these were the natural ways of handling an area of tension.

In my original pressure method, there was, however, one ramification I used which seemed rather original to me—and that was application of pressure to points on the skin by use of a pressure implement. We mentioned this briefly when describing focalization of tension at vital energy points where use of a knuckle to apply direct pressure was noticeably beneficial, but acutely tense points seemed to cry out for more specific pressure centered as precisely as possible on the point. In order to concentrate pressure more effectively, I searched for an object or implement to use, something with a diameter small enough to serve this purpose. After trying several objects, I found the best thing was the rounded end of the handle on an artist's paint brush, as shown in Fig. 1.

Acupuncture seemed perfectly logical to me upon first reading about it, since the vital energy points were what I'd been using in massage and it was understandable that piercing them would have an effect since simple massage was effective. I wasn't particularly surprised that a medical system existed which made use of points, but on doing

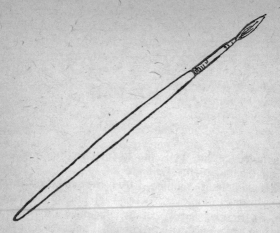

Fig. 1 Artist's brush—handle end is used to
apply acupressure

more extensive acupuncture research as background for
this book, I was startled to learn that in oriental massage
as performed by acupuncturists an implement is used to
serve the same purpose for which I was using the paint
brush handle. This tool is fashioned with a smooth,
rounded head for focusing pressure on body points. I was
a bit disappointed to read this, because I sort of thought
I'd been uniquely original and inventive in the use of the
implement. But even there, my intuition was not unique—
it was just another reiteration of intuitive discoveries that
have been made independently by persons at previous
times in history.

Again, in describing how acupressure techniques developed in my own case, we wish to impress upon you
that this method of treatment emanates from a need of
the body itself. The human system sends impulses to the
brain, impulses indicating what the system needs and what
would be beneficial to a certain condition. All members of
the animal kingdom possess this characteristic and, although some might claim that humans are an exception,
I wouldn't insult the human race by saying we don't have
such innate impulses. We do have them, but nowadays

they're usually stifled or buried by various pressures resulting from misapplication of some facets of civilization.

In the development of acupressure, my system was telling me what it needed in the way of massage to relieve tension. The method grew out of the demands of the body—it was not arbitrarily devised and superimposed on the body as something foreign, emanating from external sources. Consequently, when you sit there in your comfortable chair, rubbing muscles on your face with your thumb knuckle, or pressing certain points with the handle of a paint brush, don't let yourself feel stupid, or feel that this couldn't possibly do any good, or that it's some sort of occult ridiculousness to which some people might have had responses because they're highly suggestible and when they think they're going to have the response, they do. Suggestion often does play a role in acupuncture and acupressure effectiveness, a matter which we will consider in greater detail later on. But the power of suggestion is a strong contributing factor to the working power of all therapeutic systems, including Western medicine. And acupuncture/acupressure do work extraordinarily well without benefit of suggestion. The most commonly-mentioned proof of acupuncture's non-dependence on suggestion is its use in veterinary practice. Animals respond as successfully to acupuncture as do humans and animals are certainly not responding because of a suggestion that they do so. Acupressure massage too, being an alternate means of influencing body points, produces genuine results independent of the power of suggestion.

So—when you feel benefits, when you feel results, when you sense great improvement over a period of time—these are all real. They are as real as if you had discovered the acupressure method yourself and developed it from the needs of your own human system. They are as real as the benefits achieved during millennia of acupressure massage utilization.

33

TECHNIQUES OF ACUPRESSURE MASSAGE

A discussion of the four acupressure techniques follows:

PRESSURE

The best procedure to observe when commencing your massage is essentially the same sequence along the lines of which the method developed. Where tension is present, you'll usually have an awareness of its presence before touching the area with your hands. Let your awareness guide you—your neck may feel tight, your forehead may feel knotted, your calf muscles may feel stiff—a little rubbing with gentle pressure will then reveal the underlying tension-soreness. Continue to press and rub with your fingers or knuckles until you've located centralized tensions at the vital energy points. Always remember that pressure, whether applied by fingers, knuckles, or massage implement, should not bruise. Keep it gentle but firm. You'll sense how much pressure feels soothing and beneficial to you—don't do any more than that.

The technique is simply to press down on the vital energy point, using your knuckle or finger, with the degree of pressure that feels good, and then release. Duration of a single pressure application should usually be about ten seconds. Repeat application of pressure on the point if you like. And release. That's all there is to it.

As you work with your tensions, you'll sense when one of the points you're treating would benefit from greater centralization of pressure. Then turn to your massage implement, using it to zero in on that point. Since an artist's paint brush is probably the most readily available object meeting the requirements for use in acupressure, it's worthwhile buying one if you don't happen to have one around. A small brush isn't expensive—remember you're buying it for the handle, so the brush end can be of the most inexpensive type. Bear in mind that a short (pencil length) handle is preferable to a very long one because the shorter length is easier to use in massage—a long handle gets in the way. There are three requirements you should make certain of in the brush handle: 1) it should be of wood, plastic or other nonconductive material, 2) it should be about 1/8 inch in diameter, and 3) the handle end should be completely smooth and seamless. Some brush handles are molded in such a way as to leave a projecting seam—choose one that's totally smooth. The reason is simply that when you apply pressure to the skin, the seam may slightly scratch (break) the surface of the skin. This is not serious, the scratch would heal quickly, but we don't want to break the skin in any way with acupressure massage.

Of course in acupuncture therapy, the skin is pierced, but that's an entirely different matter—the piercing is done by skilled technicians with precision accuracy into the points, using fine needles under sterile conditions. In acupressure massage, which we do on our own, we want to avoid any breaking of the skin, so use an object that's completely smooth.

Centralization of pressure by means of the brush handle is more advantageous on some points than on others. It's particularly effective when used on the two points located where the eyebrows begin—in fact, it's generally most valuable on facial points which tend to be of a very small diameter. For neck, shoulder, and leg points, the knuckles usually provide sufficient pressure centralization since the points we use there are commonly larger. But if more precise pressure seems desirable on those points too, a good implement to use is the eraser end of a new pencil—new so that the eraser won't be worn down to where its metal holder could scratch the skin. Rubber is a nonconductor, and the eraser has no roughness which could break the skin. Such an eraser ordinarily doesn't have a rounded tip, but since neck, shoulder and leg points are larger, pressure can be effectively centralized with the eraser although it is flat. Try the eraser, try your knuckle—see which works better; use either one or alternate between them, whatever gives you the more beneficial feeling.

When employing the pressure massage technique, or

35

when using any of the other techniques described in this acupressure method, always massage only as much as feels beneficial to you. If there is any discomfort, do not continue. Discomfort isn't necessary for acupressure to be effective, in fact discomfort interferes with its effectiveness. As a general rule in applying pressure, the length of time you press down on a point should not exceed ten seconds. You'll find this is about as long as it can be maintained and remain a comforting sensation.

There's another handy tool available to all, which can be used to centralize pressure on vital energy points—that is the fingernail. When I first started pressure massage, I avoided using fingernails for fear of breaking the skin, but more recently I've learned that the nail can be used on body points with remarkable effectiveness without bruising the skin surface. When applying pressure with a nail, be especially careful to keep the pressure gentle—gentler than that applied with the knuckle or pressure implement. You'll find that in spite of its mildness, it has a distinct therapeutic effect.

Another interesting way to use fingernails is to "walk" over a tension-sore area. With the fingers flexed so that the nails hit the skin, use your index and second fingers to "walk" over the area surrounding a tense point. Observe how tension is loosened by this technique. I find fingernail "walking" most useful on the face, particularly in the high-tension areas around the eyebrows and mouth. When employing this technique, use only light pressure—again, we don't want to break the skin.

In summary, the following means of applying body point pressure are available to us: 1) using a fingertip, 2) using a knuckle, 3) use of pressure implements—paint brush handle or eraser end of a pencil, and 4) use of a fingernail. Each one is effective. Which to use at a given time is determined by which feels most beneficial to you at that time. If a pressure method such as the brush handle feels uncomfortable or excessive on a particular point, switch to one of the less potent means like a knuckle.

Before closing our discussion of the pressure technique, we must insert this word of caution: do not try acupuncture—piercing the skin—in any way on your own. It's a specialized medical skill requiring extensive training. Any piercing of the skin could possibly open the way to infection—the skin is the body's protective covering. Also, when a body point is pierced, it must be done with great precision directly in the point. Pressure massage doesn't have to be so precise and if you feel any unpleasantness, you simply stop applying pressure with no harm done. But piercing the skin at a point becomes a vastly more complicated matter and is potentially dangerous. Don't attempt piercing—confine yourself to acupressure massage on the skin surface, which is a completely safe, easy way to reap the benefits of vital energy point manipulation. And if you think that the effectiveness of massage can't come anywhere near the effectiveness of needles, consider the fact that on children, elderly, or very debilitated persons, acupuncturists themselves use point massage instead of needles. Thus the power of point massage in ratio to needles must be substantial.

MOVEMENT

This category includes rubbing, squeezing, pinching, and kneading which are done with the fingers or knuckles. Rubbing is movement back and forth, or in one direction only, over a small area surrounding a point.

Squeezing and pinching are a lifting of skin between two fingers and application of pressure. The difference between them is that in pinching, a smaller amount of skin is lifted. This technique is noticeably effective when done at tension-sore body points.

Kneading includes the various movements of working and pressing as used in kneading a mass such as dough. It's used in the general area of a point.

FRICTION

There are two types of friction which we'll consider. The first is application of pressure to a point using a finger or knuckle, then moving the skin back and forth rapidly so that the upper layer of skin in motion applies friction to underlying surfaces. This is deep friction massage. Body points on the skin surface are merely outlets for vital energy which courses through and pervades the entire human system. Applying deep friction massage to underlying surfaces at body points is a means of reaching and influencing deeper levels of the vital energy flow.

The other type of friction is applied by scratching with a fingernail on the skin at a body point. I came across a description of this technique in recent acupuncture research and it seemed a bit far-fetched to me when reading about it. The procedure is simply to scratch the point with the nail, preferably a nail that's long enough so that the skin of the finger doesn't touch the skin on the area being scratched. By scratch, we refer here to the kind of scratching you do when you have an itch, not the kind that breaks the skin and causes a wound.

The body point is thus lightly scratched, in one direction only, the action building up a mild electrical charge which, upon reaching a certain level, discharges itself along the meridian. This, according to acupuncture theory, has a beneficial effect. I was somewhat reluctant to accept the statement that such light scratching with a fingernail could be so effective. A few hours later, while writing some letters, I found myself scratching the point just to the side of my right nostril in exactly the manner described above. There was tension in the right side of my face which centralized itself in that point. I suddenly realized I often scratch this point in just this manner, moving the finger in only one direction, toward the lip. I'd long been performing automatically the very technique which seemed incredulous to me when reading it described in words on a page.

In place of the fingernail, acupuncture therapists often use a non-conducting implement for scratching—I haven't tried this, having used only the nail. Also, my fingernail is not so long that the skin of the finger doesn't touch the surface being scratched—but the technique seems beneficial in spite of that. To adequately build up a charge, however, one would have to avoid contact between the skin of the finger and the skin of the area being scratched.

I've used this technique only peripherally, mostly just as a spontaneous action without aiming for electrical charges.

PERCUSSION

The final massage-manipulation technique for influencing vital energy at acupoints is percussion. This is done by tapping or hammering the point with a fingertip or knuckle. The action is performed from a distance of two to three inches and an individual point is tapped no more than three or four times in one session. As a rule, follow your own feeling—if only one tap on a point feels like enough, let it be one—if you feel like doing three or four, then do them. Here, as with the other techniques, the amount of manipulation a point can take depends on how much tension-soreness is present. A very sore point can take only a little. As it becomes more relaxed, it can be manipulated to a greater extent.

The amount of pressure with which you hammer or tap must be controlled and, as always, pressure is determined on the basis of what feels beneficial. Start with a light tap, then increase pressure if you feel it'd be advantageous. The stronger the pressure, the fewer the number of times a point should be tapped. If tapping causes any unpleasantness or discomfort, lighten the pressure, or move to another point, or discontinue the action in favor of another technique.. There is no need to suffer any discomfort for acupressure to work. Gently does it.

Tapping may also be done with the heal of the hand, in which case a somewhat larger area surrounding the point is hit along with the point. This technique is pretty good for use on the forehead.

After tapping points, leave them alone for several days before doing it again. This is to give the area a chance to adjust to the relaxation resulting from percussion.

SUMMARY

All massage techniques are effective. We've found that, for relaxation purposes, acupressure massage may be applied in whatever manner or combination feels good to you at the time.

Although all techniques are valuable, the application of pressure precisely on the point has a unique and particularly powerful effectiveness. This technique is, however, most beneficially used in combination with other techniques rather than as the sole method employed. That is to say, the powerful effect of point pressure is most beneficial when tempered and supplemented by such manipulations as squeezing, tapping and rubbing.

SIMPLICITY OF PROCEDURE

A major characteristic of acupressure massage is its utter simplicity. In our technological society, many of us are inclined to think that something which is very simple could not possibly bring worthwhile results. This is partly due to propaganda—those to whom the promotion of technology is financially advantageous will deny the possibility that anything simple and nontechnological can have worthwhile benefits.

We certainly do not decry technology, its contributions are undeniable. We merely take issue with the rather frequently encountered attitude that nontechnological procedures are worthless or of negligible value.

The fact is that even in a field such as medicine where technology has made a substantial percentage of its greatest contributions, many simple, hand-performed procedures are still used because they work best. Such procedures are particularly impressive in medicine because they're often performed while doctor and patient are surrounded by complex equipment costing millions. A few years back, I saw films on methods of dealing with cardiac arrest. The patient is in the hospital being given emergency treatment when his heart stops beating. Immediately, closed-chest cardiac massage is performed. This is the technique where a doctor applies pressure to the patient's heart by using the heal of his hand reinforced by his other hand. Vertical pressure is applied just below med-sternum, the pressure being sufficient to depress the breast-bone an inch or a little more. It's then quickly released. This is done 60 to 70 times per minute. Probably all of you have seen the technique performed on television medical shows—it makes for a very dramatic scene since it's exciting indeed to have a doctor-actor manually mas-sage a patient's heart back to normal function while all the expensive medical machinery stands around watching him.

This simple pressure massage is what's done when the heart stops beating. So don't look upon massage as some-thing "too simple to have any worthwhile effect".

As you practice relaxation, you'll observe for yourself how even the most uncomplicated manipulation has far-reaching effects on the human mechanism. You'll see that your entire system is an intricately intertwined complex—a minor action on one part affects all other parts, some more extensively than others. You'll observe that massag-ing tense points in your calf muscles makes muscles in your face noticeably relax. And applying pressure to points on your neck makes your hands become loose and relaxed. You'll never again think "How can such a minor action do any good".

PRESENTATION SEQUENCE

In discussing acupressure as applied to various parts of the anatomy, the first segment will deal with the face. We'll talk about the key area of the forehead where point massage relieves tension over the head and down the back of the trunk, corresponding with the routes of several meridians. Then we'll consider the lower part of the face, especially around the mouth. Massage here effectively re-lieves tension down the front of the trunk, particularly relaxing the digestive and reproductive systems. This also coincides with the routes of several meridians.

41

In the second segment, we'll begin with the neck, then move to the shoulders, along the arms, and down to the fingertips. Massage of neck points promotes relaxation right into the fingers.

The third segment will deal with the legs. Massage of individual points on the legs effectively relaxes the entire legs while promoting relaxation up through the trunk and into the head. Spheres of influence of neck, arm and leg points coincide with traditional meridians.

With the exception of the face, only a few acupressure points are given for each part of the body. The reason is that only a few are needed. The entire body is, however, quite densely covered with points and many of these will, from time to time, become sore as a result of tension—any such points which you find may be treated by using the same acupressure techniques. The few points specifically discussed are major points and are usually involved when stress/tension reactions take place. Others may or may not be involved depending on the location and nature of the tension. There's no need to restrict acupressure to the points given; on the other hand, treatment of these points alone usually provides quite thorough relief of tension.

ACUPRESSURE APPLIED TO THE FACE

Our primary reason for acupressure facial massage is relaxation, both relaxation of the face muscles and the overall physical and mental relaxation which occurs simultaneously. This results in general reduction of anxiety/tension which lessens unnecessary wear and tear on the human system and improves mental and physical performance.

However, from our facial relaxation, we'll reap other welcome rewards. It we're old enough for tension to have begun showing in the face (and with some people, this begins in their twenties), acupressure massage will result in a more relaxed, attractive face with reduced wrinkling from pressure lines and avoidance of the look of aging caused by chronic muscular contractions pulling the face in distorted directions. We will, in actuality, be giving ourselves a face lift without surgery, a face lift accomplished through relaxation of those tensions which pull the face into that aged anxiety-ridden expression.

This may be of greater interest to women than men since such expression fixations as a furrowed brow are thought to make a man look intense, intelligent and mature; whereas, on a woman, they're thought of as just making her look old. Nonetheless, many men are also concerned with a youthful appearance as is evidenced, for one thing, by the considerable amount of cosmetic plastic surgery performed on men. Consequently, we shall talk about the appearance-improving aspects of facial massage as being intended for both men and women. Regardless of your sex, if retaining or achieving the look of youthful vitality is important to you, it's necessary to relax any underlying facial tensions.

The muscles in the face experience very frequent use, which is as it should be. Use is contraction (tension). But between contractions, the muscles should return to relaxation and it's when contractions become chronic that they usually develop into an entrenched expression situation. The problem, actually, is more than just that fixed, anxious facial expression, because tension manifestations in the face are indications of tensions within the human system—they're not isolated external conditions which serve only to distort your face. And the main purpose in our system of relieving facial tension is to relax the corresponding psychic and physical anxiety/tensions throughout the human system.

It is, of course, valuable to most people that they look as good as possible and this is of proven psychological significance, but improved appearance is only a bonus, so to speak, of acupressure. Our major concern is not what the tensions are doing to a person's appearance but what they're doing to his ability to function fully, and the extent to which tense muscles are unnecessarily burning fuel (energy) in order to maintain their state of tension. This burning of fuel which accomplishes no useful purpose is a needless drain on the reserves of the human system.

Naturally, there'll be many among you who have excessive/unnecessary/chronic tensions which do not presently show in the face as fixed expressions. The major such group will consist of young people among whom facial contractions have usually not yet become fixed. A second group consists of persons who are simply constructed genetically in such a way that their tensions don't settle in their faces and such persons live into rather advanced years with an essentially smooth, serene countenance although they may suffer severe anxiety/tension with serious complications elsewhere in their systems (in the form of ulcers, colitis and such). These individuals may decide facial acupressure is unnecessary since their tensions don't show. But it's the internal tensions with which we're concerned, and these may be very strong in underlying muscles where soreness can easily be felt upon applying light pressure. When such is the case, it's importance to relieve the tensions in order to achieve increased well-being and top performance capacities. I was myself quite young when I began acupressure and chronic facial expressions were definitely not my reason for doing it. My forehead felt tight and I rubbed it, discovering tense, sore muscles—and I sensed that general tensions were interfering with my ability to function at optimum levels. I started to massage those sore muscles in an effort to reduce tension. And it worked.

Among those who have developed chronic tension expressions, different persons will find they've concentrated their tensions in different areas of their faces. Some people, in nervous anxiety, constantly raise their eyebrows and soon have a network of lines over the forehead. Others maintain a stiff, tight jaw, clenching and grinding their teeth in unrelenting anxiety/tension, even while sleeping. It's noteworthy that this is a surprisingly frequent cause of loosening and eventual loss of teeth—certainly one very good reason to work on relaxing such chronic tension. Still other people frown until they have permanent, heavy, deep crevices between the brows. And what we call laugh lines aren't always caused solely by laughing, they're sometimes due to the chronic tension of maintaining a perpetually "pleasant" expression, which is as much a nervous manifestation as the fixed frown or the constant raising of eyebrows. All reveal a lack of going back to "neutral".

Neutral is the face in a state of zero repose. Serene composure should be the condition of the face between contractions. If you study a six-month old baby's face when expressing emotion and when quiet, you'll see how it shifts from extremes of expression into relaxation. All muscular contractions are released when in repose. A return to this kind of repose is what we're striving for. What happens in life is that, as a result of repeated or continuous stresses/anxieties, the face becomes fixed in one or several contractions. The frown becomes fixed. The jaw remains clenched. The raised eyebrow and tight lips become permanent. Or the artificial smile becomes glued in place.

To show yourself how tension may become fixed in the face, you might try the following: sometime when you're concentrating intently on something—taking an exam, trying to solve a difficult problem, or when you're in a business meeting determined to persuade others that your marketing approach is the correct one,—stop for a few seconds and note what contractions your efforts have caused in your facial muscles. You may have set your mouth, pulling the corners out and down with tension passing down into the jawline. You may have clenched your brows so as to cause an intricate pattern of ridges and lines to appear on your forehead. When you find yourself facing any sort of task with intense determination, stop a moment and note in what positions you've set your face. If the contractions you observe should become chronic, you'd have a tension problem showing in your face. Instead of a single stress episode, a person may go through a period of extended stress/anxiety in life, which manifests itself in certain facial contractions. Then, later, even after the stress has been eliminated, the contractions may remain because they've become habitual.

In the field of cosmetic surgery, there's much importance given to gravity as a cause of facial changes attributed to aging. The theory is that as you age, gravity pulls your skin down causing it to sag. However, it's not really gravity but loss of skin tone which causes sagging—if the skin tone remained good, gravity wouldn't make the face droop. Therefore, the health of the skin is of greater significance than age and a healthy older skin will resist the pull of gravity just about as well as a young skin. The aging process eventually causes loss of skin tone (and consequent sagging) but if a person is healthy, this shouldn't happen until very late in life.

Loss of skin tone is one reason the aged look develops too early, tension is another. In our opinion, tension is far more frequently the culprit. A vast number of the problems corrected by cosmetic facial surgery were brought about by tension. The process of aging does have some bearing on how ingrained particular tensions have become —the simple passage of years means that a fixed muscle has been maintained that much longer, therefore the contraction has become more habitual. But that muscle is not permanently tensed—it can be trained to relax again— and acupressure does exactly that. Permanent contraction is not the natural state of muscle tissue, and regardless of age, the muscle can be coaxed into relaxation. Thus a more youthful appearance is "miraculously" achieved without surgery, simply by relaxing tensions.

This doesn't mean that the effects of aging can be completely avoided. Advanced age eventually brings poor skin tone and this makes skin droop. Aging is accompanied by drying of the skin and this causes lines. But a lot is attributed to aging these days which isn't really due to aging. We can stay younger longer if we recognize those things which are making us look and feel older than we should; once recognizing them, we can overcome them. There's no doubt that tension/anxiety is a major contributor toward a premature look of age. And acupressure is the most powerful means available to us for conquering our own anxiety/tension.

So far, we've talked only about facial muscular manifestations which we want to eliminate, but there are also cases where a person with a chronic expression situation

46

is very fond of his expression and has no wish to relax it. A man may like his scowl because he feels it gives his face an intensity, an aura of superior intellectual capacity, and/or a look of severity which inspires awe in the hearts of lesser mortals. A woman may be very fond of her chronic smile—wrinkles and tension lines be damned— because she feels that only this way can she present that socially desirable picture of the "pleasant person" which is her ideal. An individual may be fond of the way his lips turn up in one corner because this gives him an air of condescension toward his employees.

Anyone who is fond of a particular facial expression, or who needs it for psychological reasons, can certainly keep it—relaxation takes place only if the person wants it to take place. Even when you massage a muscle for relaxation, if you consciously or subconsciously wish to maintain the contraction bringing about a particular expression, that contracted muscle will not relax. The will is stronger than the massage. One has to realize, however, that in order to keep a favorite expression, some amount of tension in the system must remain to maintain the required contractions, although an otherwise thorough relaxation can be achieved. Actually, as a person attains progressively better relaxation, he often loses any need to hang on to a chronic facial contraction—the relaxation resolves the psychological quirk which generated this need. But, in the meanwhile, we wouldn't want to deprive anyone of a favorite expression in the process of relieving his general anxiety/tension. After all, where would that famous actor be without his scowl?

LOCATING FACIAL TENSIONS

Although preliminary massage to locate tense acupoints may be done with either fingertips or knuckles, we personally prefer knuckles because they're smooth (there's no fingernail to get in your way while rubbing) and they give you better pressure control. The thumb knuckle is good—bend the thumb as shown in Fig. 2. Or make a loose fist with your hand and use the knuckle of the index finger. Press and rub gently all over the face. You'll find sore muscles where your tensions predominate and the pressure points in these areas will feel remarkably tender. You'll sense the difference between sensation in the surrounding muscle area and sensation at the body point.

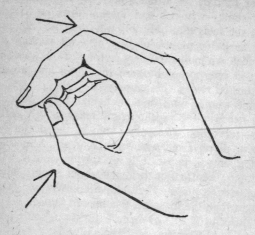

Fig. 2   Knuckle of thumb or finger may be used
for acupressure

Even if you don't have overt signs of facial tension, a light massage will locate any sore muscles and tender points, thereby revealing the amount of underlying tension which may be present. But if you do have fixed expressions, you can use them to know your major sites of tension. Like chronic stiffening of the upper lip. The saying "keep a stiff upper lip" means literally that—in trying circumstances where determination and supreme effort are required, the upper lip becomes stiffened with tension as the body rallies its forces toward conquest of the enemy, whoever or whatever that may be. This is fine for as long as circumstances demand, but becomes problematic if the stiff upper lip remains fixed in that position, never to go into relaxation again.

Thus, if you have areas with chronic expression situations, that's where your greatest concentrations of tension are likely to be. Massage those areas with your knuckles and note the acupoints. Also, try using a small mirror during some of your acupressure sessions since it helps to see the tension in your face as well as to locate it by palpation. Usually, we've lived with our tensions for so long, we're only vaguely aware that the face is being pulled into fixed expressions, which are maintained unconsciously, and a mirror can make us face these little facts. However, it's well known that before looking in a mirror, we spontaneously relax our faces as best we can so as to look as good as possible to ourselves. So we have to trick ourselves a little. Do this by taking a few minutes during an acupressure session to sit quietly with a small mirror in your hand just looking at your face. Don't stare, just look at it casually. If chronic expression tendencies are strong inclinations in your facial muscles, your "mirror expression" will slowly leave and your usual tensions creep back in. You'll observe the muscles pulling your eyebrows into a frown, dragging the corners of the mouth down, raising the brows to create a lined forehead, or whatever. When you see this taking place, you know where to concentrate your acupressure efforts.

ACUPRESSURE POINTS ON THE FACE

Fig. 3 is a diagrammatic illustration showing important acupoints on the face, as well as directions in which tension pulls muscles to bring about the strained expressions contributory toward an aged look.

All the tension manifestations indicated are natural muscular movements (contractions) which take place when facial expressions and/or muscular reactions to stress occur. The contractions (tensions) become problematic only when they become chronic, when the muscles do not return to relaxation after the expression and/or stress reaction has passed.

Of the various major tensions illustrated, an individual may present any one or any combination in his/her face. Other chronic contractions may also occur, although these are the most common.

Arrows indicate the directions in which tensions usually pull. Large black circles signify major pressure points,

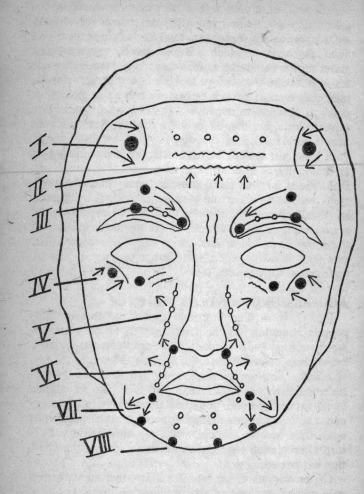

Fig. 3 Acupressure points on the face. Roman numerals refer to descriptive paragraphs in the text

50

the manipulation of which is exceedingly effective in reducing tension. Smaller white circles are additional valuable points to massage. The positions of points in the
illustration are approximate since exact locations depend
on the individual shape and size of your own face and
features. Use the drawing as a guide to help you determine
point locations, bearing in mind that your face is unique
and points may not be quite where they are in the dia-
gram. (The same holds true for points anywhere on your
body—use the diagrams in this book as a guide; use
palpation to locate precise positions of points on your
own body.)

A brief description of each tension manifestation shown
in Fig. 3 follows:

I. These tensions pull inward and somewhat downward
to aggravate crease marks between the brows. To demonstrate this to yourself, rest a finger lightly on the area of the
acupoint—then pull your eyebrows together vigorously in
a strong frown. Note how the muscles under your finger
are pulling inward and slightly downward.

II. Many people raise their eyebrows in chronic nervous
tension which results in a furrowed brow, sometimes with
and sometimes without the addition of a frown.

III. These muscles pull inward to cause crease marks
between the eyebrows. This fixation, the frown, is perhaps
the most common of chronic facial contractions.

IV. Tension pulls these muscles inward and upward to
accentuate wrinkles under the eyes. Squinting, which often
becomes a tension manifestation, is partly accomplished
by means of these contractions. The indicated vital energy
point is located on the cheekbone and is often tender due
to tension.

The point shown directly below the center of the eye is
a powerful acupoint for general relaxation use. This one
has point sensation and most of you will be able to feel
it on applying pressure.

V. These muscles pull sideways and slightly upwards
to accentuate wrinkles under the eyes, working also to
pull the tip of the nose down.

VI. These muscles pull sideways and somewhat upwards to make crease marks, also pulling the tip of the nose down. Men aren't usually concerned with the contour of their nose-tips, but on women, a drooping nose-tip is generally considered a primary contributory factor toward an aged look. Plastic surgeons consistently raise nose-tips to give a semblance of youth. Drooping nose-tips are attributed to several causes other than tension, but we believe tension is a major cause, if not the major one. It's chronic muscular contractions at the sides of the nose pulling outward and upward that causes the nose-tip to droop. If you want to demonstrate this to yourself, simply place your index fingers flat along the two tension lines leading from nose to mouth, with fingertips on the acupoints just below the nostrils. Then push inward and slightly downward—you'll see your tip-of-the-nose contour raise itself while your upper lip also becomes relaxed. The foregoing assumes, of course, that you have tension in this area of your face—if it's relaxed, then it already presents its natural contour.

VII. These muscles pull down to draw the corners of the mouth downward and contribute toward formation of the sagging contour illustrated in Fig. 4, a common occur-

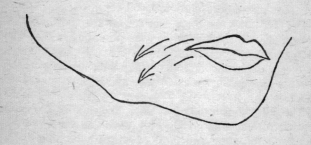

Fig. 4 The bulging jawline

rence among older people. A friend who had developed this contour attributed it to the years and to slight weight gain. However, after practicing acupressure facial massage over a period of several months for the purpose of general relaxation, she found this bulging contour had vanished, and her jawline was again as smooth as it had been years previously. She had lost no weight and certainly hadn't lost any years, therefore she concluded the bulge must have been caused by tension. Tight muscles were pulling down at the corners of the mouth and created the droop in the jawline. We believe this is often the case—it's not age as much as loss of muscle flexibility through chronic tension that causes these droops to appear. A relaxed face will retain its youthful contour numerous years longer than one distorted by chronic muscular contractions.

VIII. These muscles often become tension-sore when general mouth tension is severe. If this occurs, the acupoints indicated will be sore on pressure and are valuable points for massage.

The "miracle" of suddenly looking years younger—it can be yours through the simple process of relaxation. Chronic tension forces the face into fixed contractions, thereby creating an appearance of advanced age. If you have such tension and you succeed in releasing the musculature, your face will resume its smooth, serene mien of repose and immediately look many years younger. Don't be surprised if you suddenly observe that people with whom you have casual contact, such as salespersons, bank personnel, waiters, etc, who previously behaved toward you as if you were an "older, mature" customer now behave as if they believe you to be much younger. People who know you well, on the other hand, may ask incredulously "what are you doing, taking 'get younger' pills?", or they may simply admire you in envious silence.

If a more youthful appearance were the sole benefit we reaped from acupressure relaxation, it would be well worth the time. But the benefits are vastly greater; indeed, they are of truly remarkable proportions.

PREPARATION FOR ACUPRESSURE

Before doing acupressure, always wash your hands well with soap and water. It is, in fact, good to do the massage within a few hours after showering or bathing so there's a minimum of debris on your skin, either in the form of waste matter emitted from the body (perspiration, accumulated oils, etc.) or dust, soot, germs, etc. picked up from the environment.

Do not apply oil to the skin before doing acupressure massage. Traction is needed for this type of massage, an oily surface is too slippery.

If you like, you might apply a little mild antiseptic to your fingers for added cleanliness before starting acupressure. A little tincture of iodine rubbed over each fingertip and nail is good—iodine stains your skin slightly but that wears off within an hour or so. Or some hydrogen-peroxide (antiseptic 3%), or alcohol on the fingertips is nice. Fingers are our major contact with the environment, touching everything from money to doorknobs, and fingernails have crevices where bacteria picked up during a day's worth of living could hide from soap and water. A little antiseptic after washing provides enhanced cleanliness before using your fingers on your skin, and it's particularly good when performing any massage techniques done with the fingernail.

When you do acupressure, give yourself plenty of time to spend on it. Don't feel nervous about taking the time, don't feel guilty because you think there are other, more important things you should be doing. There's very little that's more important than your relaxation and well-being. So give yourself enough time, at least a half hour. You'll find yourself functioning so much better in all your pursuits after your tensions have started melting away that it'll become progressively easier to persuade yourself to take the time for acupressure.

Start by sitting down in a comfortable chair. Your back and head should be supported by the back of the chair and your legs elevated on a footstool. You should be seated in such a way that you can let go of your entire musculature, so that you don't have to contract any muscles to support, or maintain the position of, any part of your body. Now close your eyes. Let your lungs go. Drop them as if you intended for them to fall right to the floor. Let them breathe naturally—you don't have to make lungs breathe, they do so of their own accord. You'll find your lungs emptying themselves before each new breath is taken—this is in contrast to the shallow, partial breathing one does when under tension. Relaxing the lungs, of and by itself, encourages excellent general relaxation throughout the human system—which is, incidentally, the basis upon which "breathing exercises" work. But we shall proceed to do a complete step-by-step relaxation along the entire length of the body, starting at the feet (a more detailed description of this process is given in our book **Relaxation Renewal,** under "Relaxation Procedure"). Let the feet become limp and heavy as if each weighed 200 pounds. Let them sink into the footstool. Just drop them. When you've let them go as much as you can, do the same with the calves, then the thighs, working your way on up through the torso to the head. Release every voluntary contraction you can find in your body. When you've gone as limp and heavy all over as possible, stay that way a few minutes. Think of yourself as a soaking wet towel lying there draped in the chair. Now open your eyes. You're ready to begin acupressure.

ACUPRESSURE PROCEDURE

Rubbing with a knuckle is not only the best way to locate centralized tension at points, it's also the best technique with which to start massage when you've determined which points you're going to treat. Use your knuckle to rub the area of a point in different directions, varying the pressure. Do it slowly, take your time. When you press the acupoint, you'll feel the desire to relax vast areas of your musculature throughout your body—proceed to consciously follow through on that desire. Let go in every bit of muscle where you feel the inclination. Just let everything drop, as if you intended for your muscles to fall to the floor. Don't worry, they won't—although many of us

55

walk around hanging on so tensely to our innards, you'd think they would fall out if it weren't for the tight grip we keep on them.

Follow the application of pressure by trying other massage techniques—squeeze, pinch, knead, or tap the tense area. If pinching feels good, pinch—if tapping feels good, tap. Remember that it's our intention to do massage which feels soothing and relaxing, using the example again of having someone squeeze and rub tense muscles in the back of your neck at the shoulders. The maxim to follow in acupressure is: always be gentle and pursue the action only if it feels beneficial to you. If a point or muscle area is unusually tension-sore, do just a little, soft massage until some relaxation has taken place, then you can do more.

Working the various tension-sore spots on your face with fingers and knuckles may be the only kind of massage manipulation that's needed. But if certain points feel as if they'd benefit from more centralized pressure, then use the brush handle. Since tensions focalize themselves in points, applying pressure precisely on them has a substantially more powerful effect than generalized massage of the area. Some of the most useful spots for centralizing pressure are the points where the eyebrows begin, the point at the arch of each eyebrow, points on the cheekbone, at the side of each nostril, at the corners of the mouth and bottom of the chin. These are indicated as solid black in Fig. 3. When using the brush handle as a massage implement, hold the brush as you normally would, but with the handle end down. Apply slight pressure, moving the handle around in the immediate vicinity of the point. When you've located the exact spot where tension soreness is centralized, you'll recognize it by the sensation. Then press down with gentle but firmer pressure on that spot. Hold for several seconds—no more than ten. And release. You'll sense the effect this has on your system. If you wish, press down again for several seconds and release. You might do it a third time, but no more than three times on a single point in one acupressure session. Occasionally, you may want to vibrate the implement rapidly back and forth, or up and down, while applying pressure on the point—this produces enhanced effect.

Sometimes you'll want to press a single acupoint only once, and then go on to other points, while at other times, you'll prefer two or three applications of pressure on each. The amount you do will usually depend on how much tension you find in the spot, revealed by how sore it is. If it's very sore, apply pressure only once, then come back to it several days later. If it's moderately sore, you can apply pressure two or three times. On a slightly tense point, you can apply the amount of pressure you feel helpful, maybe once, maybe more often. Pressure has its greatest effect on points presenting extreme tension soreness, although these can't take too much treatment and must be handled with care. As they become relaxed, they can take a lot more treatment but it won't have as powerful an effect since the amount of tension present is much less than before. After tension in an area has been substantially worked out over a period of time, precision pressure applied with the brush handle is not necessary and you won't get the same feeling of relief when you apply it. When such is the case, simple knuckle massage is adequate. Again, go by what you feel. After locating a tense point, try a finger or knuckle on it and see if it feels sufficient. If yes, stay with that. If you need more pressure, use the brush handle.

When you've become adept at locating points and controlling pressure, you may wish to try using your fingernail (index finger is best). This pressure must be lighter than that applied with an implement, so as not to cut the skin. Limit the application to five seconds on a point, otherwise follow the same guidelines as when using an implement. You might also try vibrating a fingernail rapidly back and forth on the point—but make certain the pressure is especially gentle when you're doing this. "Fingernail walking", as described in the section on massage techniques, is another valuable variation, particularly when done on high tension areas. This is the technique where you flex the fingers and walk on the skin with the fingertips, permitting the nails to hit the skin with slight pressure.

In addition to pressure and movement manipulations (rubbing, squeezing, pinching, kneading), you should try deep friction and tapping. The latter is especially beneficial on forehead points, not so much on lower face points. Deep friction is good in most areas of tension on the face.

There's no need to use all techniques in any one session —you may want to use only one or two. In a later session, you may use entirely different techniques. You know when something feels good to you and that's all you need as your guideline—use the technique that feels beneficial and do as much manipulation as feels beneficial.

If you have an illness, you might experience a different effect from massage, other than simple relaxation. Should you find acupressure disturbing, uncomfortable or aggravating in any way, discontinue it. Don't massage a point which is spontaneously painful, or exhibits any other symptoms of illness. If you have an advanced disease condition, consult a physician before doing vital energy point massage. Also, we reiterate, don't attempt piercing any body points yourself. If you have an ailment which you think might respond favorably to acupuncture, consult your physician and seek his recommendation.

SPHERES OF INFLUENCE. Surely one of its most intriguing aspects is the fact that acupressure point massage promotes relaxation along such vast spheres of influence throughout the human system due to the fact that tensions are intertwined in an intricately knit pattern. When massaging a point on the center of your cheekbone, you'll find your solar plexus relaxing. When smoothing away the tensions along your eyebrows, you'll find the tightness in back of your head subsiding. Every point will promote relaxation along a sphere of influence—no point exists in limbo all by its lonesome.

Always go with the inclination toward relaxation along spheres throughout your system when applying any of the acupressure techniques. If massaging the point at the corner of the mouth (which is on the stomach meridian) makes you want to let go of your stomach and intestines, do so. Drop them. Let all the muscles around them go loose. Keep letting go everywhere you feel the sensation to let go. Follow through on your desire to relax anywhere in the body, don't confine your relaxation to the small area where you're doing acupressure. Bear in mind that the human system doesn't consist of separate independent parts which adhere loosely together; it's an inextricably interwoven Whole with each part dependent upon and reacting to all other parts.

One of the most interesting examples of the spheres of influence is the manner in which relaxation of the mouth makes the reproduction system relax. Massage around the mouth, both general and concentrated on points, automatically relaxes the lower abdomen area, particularly the sex organs. It's almost as if a wire connects the two areas and the act of letting go around the mouth is transmitted right along that wire bringing about relaxation along its length and particularly at its opposite end in the reproductive system. In ancient Chinese medicine, the sphere of influence from the mouth down the front center of the body is a principle meridian known as the Conception Vessel Meridian. When you feel response along this vessel path, you have an ancient medical system verifying that your response is real, it's not your imagination and you're not reacting to suggestion. The sphere of influence is genuine and most useful, being an easy way to relax the entire reproductive system, thereby helping to solve numerous sexual problems which have their origins in tension.

In the above paragraphs, we've been talking about physical ramifications of relaxation achieved through influencing vital energy by means of body point manipulation. It is imperative to remember that, at the same time, the mind also becomes relaxed. Among those groups and/or civilizations which have extensively contemplated the nature of vital energy, it has been generally conceded that said energy is largely responsible for mind. For acupressure purposes, we do not need to understand how vital energy produces mind, it's sufficient for us to know that

V-energy manipulation influences the mind in the same ratio that it influences physiological functioning. Indeed, as previously stated, mind and body constitute a single entity and mental relaxation occurs simultaneously with physical relaxation. This is true not only because of vital energy's "total" influence but also because the musculature must inevitably be utilized in order for any mental process to take place. If the musculature is totally relaxed, mental processes stop.

On the other hand, if you interfere with or resist muscular relaxation, mental relaxation will not occur. Your volition is stronger than the relaxation process. If you apply acupressure and resist the relaxation, refusing to let the muscles go, you will not become relaxed. The same holds true regardless of what relaxation method you practice. If you do meditation and refuse to let go of a single muscle, you're going to emerge from your session just as tense as you were when you started. If you use biofeedback equipment and refuse to let go of the muscles where the instrument indicates you've tensed them, they'll remain tensed. None of the intellectually-oriented relaxation techniques, which are by their nature dependent upon your cooperation, will work if you refuse to let the muscles go. Such things as drugs, electric shock, or acupuncture can force relaxation; but a biofeedback instrument, meditation, or acupressure massage cannot, if you decide not to become relaxed.

Therefore, when employing acupressure, you must go with the relaxation. If out of resistance, or fear, the conscious (or subconscious) volition refuses relaxation, you will remain essentially tense. The volition must want and encourage relaxation. In acupressure, the mind and volition should be occupied almost exclusively with following through on relaxation, going with the inclination to let all the muscles hang loose along spheres of influence. Other than that, just let the mind roam freely, don't try to restrict or control it. Freedom combined with acupressure will shift your brain into either alpha or beta waves.

In pursuing acupressure, bear in mind that relaxation is simply to stop using the musculature, to just let it go.

Relaxation is not an action that you perform—it is not performing any action. Many people make an effort to relax, and twist their muscles into new tensions in this effort to overcome existing tensions. Relaxation is not an effort. Don't work at it—relaxing is the opposite of working or doing, it's doing nothing. Relaxation is accomplished by letting go, by dropping, by releasing the muscles into zero repose which means "not doing".

There's another important factor to keep in mind: if you're massaging, tapping, or applying pressure so hard that you cause your musculature to contract (tense up) against the hurt, then you're doing it too hard. Anytime you apply, anywhere on the body, sufficient pressure to cause hurt, your musculature will tense up in defense against that hurt. We don't want to cause this reaction in the muscles. Our aim is to persuade muscles to relax. Therefore, at all times, apply only enough pressure so that it's soothing and encourages relaxation, never so much that muscles contract in self-defense.

To clarify the difference between proper pressure and too much pressure, we can again use the example of having tension-sore muscles rubbed in back of the neck. If the person who's rubbing does it too hard, your reaction will be actual pain and you'll tense up against the hurt. If he rubs with the right amount of pressure, it'll be soothing and relaxing.

HOW MUCH MASSAGE YOU SHOULD DO. Perform as much acupressure as feels good, then leave it. If the muscles and body points are very sore, leave it for quite a length of time—several days or even weeks—until the body has fully absorbed and adjusted to the relaxation brought about by the massage. You can judge very easily how much to do in one session—just use the feeling in back of the lower neck. You know when the neck's been massaged enough, and after letting it rest a while, you can sense when it's ready for more. Go by these same sort of feelings when determining extent and frequency of massage anywhere else on your body.

Do not attempt to massage or apply pressure to a point until it's completely free of tension-soreness since this can-

61

not be accomplished within the period of the massage session itself. If tension in an area is extreme, the first muscular reaction to massage will be a different kind of soreness, the kind that comes when a muscle suddenly finds itself flexible and usable again after so long in a state of chronic contraction. It's in such cases that it'll take several days to a week for soreness to subside. When enough time has elapsed, the muscles will have become adjusted to their new degree of relaxation and can be relaxed some more. Additional massage will accomplish greater relaxation, and so on until zero repose, or close to it, is reached. If tension is only moderate, muscular reaction to relaxation will be less pronounced, but a period of adjustment to the newly-relaxed state will still be required. It's not until after this adjustment period that tension-soreness completely disappears from the point.

Also, you're not going to rid yourself totally of your tensions by practicing only one or two sessions of acupressure massage—or of any other kind of relaxation therapy, for that matter. It's taken your lifetime to collect the assortment of tensions you now have and you won't undo in a half hour what's taken years to accumulate. Besides, there's the fact that you continue to live between relaxation sessions and therefore continue to be subjected to stress and tension. This is a normal part of life and our aim is not to take the living out of life, but to help you become able to relax between the stresses and strains. In consequence, you'll be healthier, you'll function fully and be able to cope with life's stresses more successfully because you're using your total capabilities.

There's no need to maintain any kind of regular schedule with acupressure—like an hour each morning or 20 minutes twice a day. Do it whenever you can make the time, whether days or weeks apart. As you become more and more aware of the nature of tensions, you'll be able to recognize when they've built up inside you and will realize that you need to do some relaxation. Then give yourself an acupressure session first chance you get. On the other hand, don't wait only for severe tension conditions—do acupressure whenever the mood strikes you.

You probably won't be able to relax down to zero repose when you first start acupressure, but whatever degree of relaxation you manage to achieve within, say, a month will be noticeably beneficial. You don't need total relaxation to benefit. If your tensions are extreme and you succeed in relaxing away only 4% of those tensions during your first few acupressure sessions, the result will still be startlingly obvious to you in a calmer outlook, improved performance, and increased capacity to handle stress.

Even when you become sufficiently adept at relaxation to achieve zero repose, there'll most likely be periods in the future during which your stresses are so frequent and severe as to make it virtually impossible to relax to zero between them. Here too, whatever degree of relaxation is achieved means improved capacity to deal with forthcoming and ongoing stress.

SHAKING OF THE HEAD

Another useful aid to relaxation is shaking the head. This technique is simplicity itself—you merely turn your head rapidly from side to side. It serves as a general loosening up. It's not really acupressure but is peripheral to it in that shaking jolts vital energy and head muscles into letting go.

The procedure is as follows: close your eyes and shake your head rapidly keeping it as limp as possible. Shake first over a small radius—that is, moving only a small distance from side to side. Then shake over a larger radius, turning almost as far as the head comfortably turns without moving the shoulders (see Fig. 5). Shaking over the larger radius should be done a bit more slowly.

Shake only as many times as feels good to you. If it feels discomforting or makes you dizzy, then stop. A head that's very tense will be able to take only a few shakes back and forth, a more relaxed head enjoys being shaken a greater number of times.

After shaking, contemplate a moment and note the areas in your head that have been loosened. You'll feel a desire to consciously relax areas of the brain and down

63

the spinal cord at the back of the neck. Follow through on it.

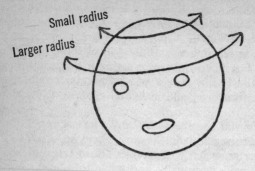

Fig. 5   Head shaking

Head shaking helps relax all systems for better overall body tone. Many meridians have spheres of influence up into and around the head; consequently, shaking breaks tension patterns in numerous body points and their spheres, engendering vital energy balance with concurrent relaxation of musculature, nervous system, etc.

VITAL ENERGY POINTS SERVE AS TIE-LINES TO INNER TENSIONS

We've already mentioned that sometimes, even among older people, tensions don't manifest themselves in chronic facial expressions, although they're very strong internally. Tensions will centralize themselves in different parts of the body in different people. John, who died at 38 of bleeding ulcers, had the smoothest, most unperturbed-appearing face imaginable. He looked as if his life was one of calm satisfaction while, inside, his stomach was being corroded by stress and anxiety. He did talk about his stresses; he worked as assistant to a hard-driving prosecuting attorney. He was well paid, but worked under unrelenting pressure. Additionally, he lived with, and was the sole support of, his elderly father, who managed to

64

keep the son from becoming seriously attached to a woman for fear of losing him to marriage and being left alone. John had suffered stomach pains but was told it was all psychological. A few weeks later he was dead.

The ulcer pain did indeed have psychological origins in stress/tension/anxiety but had long since progressed to a severe physiological illness. Again we are reminded that the human system is one, inseparable unit—psychological stresses often engender physical ailments and conversely, physical illnesses usually affect the mental state of the individual.

Physiological manifestations of psychological stress/tension/anxiety may focus themselves in the stomach, heart, large intestine (bowel), or any of several other locations. One's genetic makeup seems to have some bearing on where tensions will be inclined to focus in an individual. But, although tension may choose to centralize itself in an internal organ, it will be reflected in numerous areas of the musculature and in body points. A little gentle pressing and rubbing reveals the tension-soreness in these areas and points. Simple massage of the points can then relieve the inner tensions.

Thus, although chronic expression contractions may not be obvious in the face, inner tensions will nevertheless reflect themselves in point soreness on the face and elsewhere on the body. It behooves us to take advantage of these tie-lines with our inner tensions, these vital energy points which provide us with an easy, yet amazingly powerful means of relaxing our internal tensions through simple massage.

ACUPRESSURE APPLIED TO THE NECK, SHOULDERS, ARMS, HANDS

FRONT OF NECK AND SHOULDERS

Key points on the neck and upper shoulders are extraordinarily effective in relaxing the entire arms and hands right down to the fingertips. Fig. 6 shows two

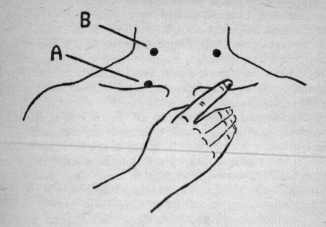

Fig. 6   Front-of-neck points

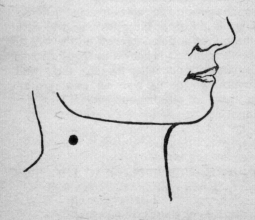

Fig. 7   Side-of-neck point

unusually powerful vital energy points on the front of the neck. Even when there's no chronic tension condition present, pressure on point A usually produces not only point sensation but a certain amount of sensation along the meridian leading down the arm. If tensions are present in the arm and hand, the effect of acupressure on this neck point is especially strong, and the path of influence can be felt forcefully right down into the fingers.

To locate point A on your neck, sit comfortably relaxed in a chair. Place a fingertip at your collarbone (clavicle) about two inches from the knob as shown in Fig. 6. It's best to use your right hand on the left collarbone point and vice versa, so that the arm responding to point pressure is free to become loose and relaxed. The acupoint is close to and almost behind the bone, and its position can be precisely determined by applying pressure.

Now move your finger upwards along your neck about 1 1/2 inches. Feel around and you'll find another pressure spot that has point sensation, which is point B in Fig. 6. If you press it when there's great tension in your arm and hand, you'll feel remarkable soreness down the entire sphere of influence right into the hand.

Pressure is the most effective massage technique on both of these points. First, apply gentle pressure with your finger, moving it around slightly so the upper layer of skin moves over underlying tissues. In this way, you can zero in on the exact nucleus of the point. Then, holding the finger still, apply slightly greater pressure directly on the point. Rub the point area a little too, then lift up and squeeze the skin between your fingers, always consciously encouraging the head, neck, arms, etc. to relax as much as possible.

There's also an excellent point toward the side of the neck, located about midway between head and shoulder (see Fig. 7). Let's say your right side is tension-sore— then you'll probably feel soreness sensation all the way up over that side of your head and into the ocular region above the right eye when you press this point. At the same time, if the left side is relaxed, you'll feel nothing but normal point sensation there. Several months ago, when

I had tension on the right side of my head and applied pressure to this point, I could feel soreness sensation all along the meridian up over the head and into the eyebrow. However, when I pressed the same point on the left side, I got only point sensation. Today the tension is gone and I get only point sensation on both sides of the neck. To remove the tension, I had applied pressure with my knuckle plus some with the eraser head of a new pencil. Also did a little movement massage of the area, all of which felt quite beneficial.

The three points discussed above seem to be the most potent for acupressure in this region of the neck. However, there are many which may become tender and therefore locatable when tension-soreness is present—otherwise they have no sensation. If you come upon such tense points, take the time to press and massage those. Use any combination of techniques with the exception of percussion (tapping) which is not particularly beneficial in this area.

As you proceed to apply acupressure to tense neck points, remind yourself that although it may seem "something this simple can't possibly do any good", it does do good, and over a period of time, you'll be aware of the good. But remember also that since the neck is an area where chronic tension notoriously enjoys settling, it's going to creep back in rather readily and you may be massaging there often. However, as you make progress in relaxation techniques, you'll find yourself able to consciously relax the neck more easily when it's tense and you'll automatically fall into a more relaxed state between the inevitable stress/tension situations of living.

The fact that relaxation is not permanent does not mean relaxation doesn't work—it simply means you're alive and consequently subject to stresses, strains, and anxieties on a continuing basis, which means tensions may become reestablished in your system. There's nothing wrong with tensions, they're a normal part of living. But when a stress/tension episode has passed, we should return to relaxation, and it's the unnecessary/chronic/excessive tension which often remains that becomes a problem. The important thing is: don't think that because tensions reappear, the relaxation method isn't working. Our modern technological life-style is such that persuading our systems to relax between stresses is usually a life-long occupation. The pressures of living are so pervasive that the tendency is to live a chronically tense existence, and when a brief respite of relaxation is achieved, the tensions are exceedingly eager to rush right back in. We must therefore faithfully continue practicing relaxation techniques, since this is the means by which we can successfully avoid succumbing to a life ridden with unnecessary tension with its accompanying detriments such as needless drain on our energy resources, blockage of our creative potential, and attrition of our good health.

BACK OF NECK AND SHOULDERS

Tension/anxiety manifests itself powerfully in the forehead, up over the head, and down through the back of the neck. We need only consider that headache is probably the most frequent overt symptom of anxiety/tension and we realize the importance of this area in the expression of tension. Numerous vital energy points on the forehead, the head, and back of the neck will become sensitive under stress. We talked about forehead points in the section on face massage—many of the same points involved in facial tension-contractions will also become tension-sore in headache. In addition, other points will present soreness—they can easily be located by palpation. Indeed, if you've been under severe stress which has brought on a splitting headache, you may find what seems an endless number of sore points on the forehead as well as all over the top of the head.

In tension-headache, forehead points may be treated with gentle pressure and careful massage—their extreme sensitivity necessitates special tenderness in handling. As for the scalp points, we've usually found they quiet down of their own accord when forehead and back-of-neck points are massaged. We've occasionally used some pres-

69

sure and light tapping on top-of-head points, but basically they've been left alone knowing they'd respond to forehead and back-of-neck treatment.

At the junction of the head and back-of-neck is located an especially famous point of soreness in headache—point C in Fig. 8. Many Western masseurs, although not cognizant of acupuncture theory, know this point and recognize the manner in which it mirrors headache. There'll no doubt be other tension-sensitized points around the base of the skull—wherever you find soreness, treat it with acupressure.

Pressure on point C is so valuable in relieving head and neck tension that we'd like to suggest an alternate way of applying it. Locate a high-backed chair with a hard, smooth, rounded edge at the top of the back. The edge should be at a height which makes it possible to position the base of your skull against it as in Fig. 9. After placing your head as illustrated, push against the edge so as to apply pressure to the point area. Continue doing so for several seconds, as long as it feels beneficial. Then move the head and press any other points which may be tension-sore. It's also important to use the other massage techniques on these points, namely rubbing, squeezing and applying pressure by hand with the eraser end of a pencil. The eraser works really well—if you prefer, it can do the job in lieu of a high-backed chair.

The overwhelming frequency with which tension-headache afflicts human beings in today's living environment is one of the more obvious indications of the incessant stress under which so many of us subsist. Acupressure relaxation techniques can effectively resolve stress-tension headache, but in addition to doing the acupressure, you must also be willing to give yourself the time necessary to untangle your knotted muscles and you must remove yourself, at least temporarily, from the situation which is inflicting excessive stress on you. In other words, if the stress/tension headache is being caused by a trying business crisis, the headache won't be cured just by pressing a few choice body points. You must detach yourself from your stress situation, drop into a comfortable chair,

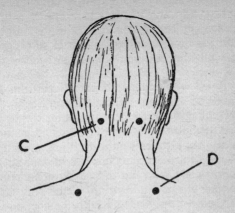

Fig. 8 Back-of-neck and shoulder points

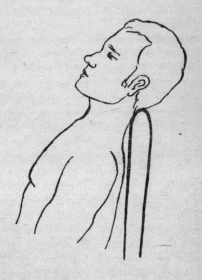

**Fig. 9 Positioning of neck against back of chair in order
to apply pressure**

71

separate yourself from the problems which are causing the twisted, knotted muscles now throbbing in your head. Then gently and easily, you can pressure-massage your head and back-of-neck points. Let go of all those tightly-contracted muscles and your tension headache will soon vanish.

The reason relaxation techniques performed while you're involved in a stress situation won't cure a tension headache is that the cause is still present. Unless you can manage to completely let go of your musculature while under stress—an extremely difficult, if not impossible, task since tension naturally occurs concurrent with stress—you cannot completely free yourself of tension-caused pain. But a moment or two of relaxation, even if only superficial, can nevertheless help you cope with the continued stress. Therefore, to take a few seconds now and then, while under stress, for application of acupressure on head points and some releasing of the musculature won't remove your headache but will make it easier for you to cope with the ongoing crisis/stress.

It's important to recognize that the manner in which relaxation resolves a headache is quite different from how drugs resolve it. An analgesic drug blocks the pain impulses being emitted by knotted, tightly contracted muscles, whereas relaxation removes the pain by removing the contractions. (Bear in mind that we're dealing with tension/ stress/anxiety-caused headache—numerous other conditions such as tumors or meningitis will also bring on headache which cannot, of course, be cured with simple relaxation. The vast majority of headaches are, however, tension-caused.) Analgesics—such as aspirin—will relieve headache while you are under ongoing stress since the drug blocks pain impulse, therefore doesn't require removal of cause. Often tranquilizers are given along with an analgesic, in recognition of tension's role in pain, and tranquilizers can (depending on the type) bring about some muscular relaxation. They also make you drowsy, dull your concentration, and generally make it difficult to work. Thus, how you relieve stress/tension headache would depend on the stress situation and what it demands of you. In general, the easiest, safest relief is relaxation. And the most potent, efficient means of achieving relaxation is acupressure.

During the course of this book, when describing how tension-soreness feels, we've often made reference to how muscles in back of the neck and upper shoulders feel when tense. We all know tension is inordinately fond of ensconcing itself in this area and are familiar with the tight, knotted sensation. A major reason the large muscles at the back and sides of the neck are so extraordinarily prone to tension is the fact they they work to hold the head up. A person is so accustomed to their being in use that he may not even be aware muscle power is involved, assuming the head sort of stays up by itself. All you need do in order to illustrate use of these muscles is to sit in a chair holding your head normally, then let it go, just let every muscle in your neck relax completely, letting your head become loose like a blob. Observe how it drops forward when the muscles are released. Since these neck muscles are in virtually constant use during waking hours, tension can creep in and remain there with the person almost unaware of its presence. It often becomes so much an integral part of a person that even during sleep, when these muscles would normally be released, they remain in a predominantly tensed state with only a superficial relaxation taking place as the head is laid on the pillow.

After we've successfully achieved a degree of relaxation in the neck and upper shoulders, tension will be so eager to return that it'll be necessary to monitor these muscles constantly and persuade them back into relaxation whenever they become knotted with contractions. It's our aim to relieve these and all similar tensions throughout the body. What we want to achieve is to have the head held up with only that amount of muscle power necessary to hold it up, thus avoiding the wear and tear of using excess muscle power (the situation caused by accumulation of excessive/unnecessary/chronic tension). And we want to reach the state where, when the head hits the pillow at night, the neck will, of its own accord, fall into an optimum relaxation. Ditto for the rest of the body.

73

A bit below the neck, at the back of the shoulders (point D in Fig. 8), you'll find another valuable point on which the fingers or pencil eraser may be used. If you have someone who'll do acupressure for you, this is a spot where he/she could be helpful since this is one place where it's nice to have someone else massage you. A wife or husband is always an excellent person to call on as a personal masseur, but anyone is useful as long as he/she is willing to learn a little about point massage, and agrees to be serious when doing it. Many people (Americans especially) tend to think of massage as either humorous or sexy—it's not thought to be a therapeutic factor worthy of serious consideration. Massage, then, is quickly turned into either a joke or a seduction scene. Jokes and seductions are delightful, of course, but they're not what we're aiming for in this acupressure method.

If you have someone who'll do a little serious back massage for you, that's fine, but we're of the opinion that anywhere on the body except the back, it's better for a person to do his own acupressure. The primary reason is, as we've stated before, that you can monitor your responses at all times, and adjust your massage accordingly. You can even do a very good job on the back of your own neck and upper shoulders if someone else isn't available. As for points toward the center of your back which are beyond your reach for acupressure purposes, massage in this area isn't required since excellent total relaxation is achieved by working key areas within your reach. You'll observe that applying acupressure on the forehead, and back of the neck will relax your entire back right down to your buttocks. This is certainly logical when we consider that several meridians—including the Governor Vessel Meridian which passes down the center of the back directly on the spine—have spheres of influence extending from the forehead, up over the head, and down the back.

NECK STRETCHING
Stretching the neck muscles also serves to relax your back as well as the neck. This, like head-shaking, is not

really an acupressure technique, but is a valuable adjunct to it. Stretching is as ridiculously simple as shaking and is equally effective.

If you drop your head to the right side, as far down toward the shoulder as it'll go, you'll feel the muscles stretch on the left. They may feel sore, the amount of soreness depending on the amount of tension in the muscles. While letting your head hang there dropped toward your shoulder, move it back and forth a ways, bob it up and down a little—as you're doing this, just let go of everything and give in to the stretch.

The act of stretching is very relaxing to the human system. People used to do a lot more of it—when awakening from sleep, for example. But with those ubiquitous alarm clocks and hurry-up tensions goading us all the time, many of us have buried away somewhere our natural instinct to stretch simply because "there's no time".

The principle of stretch is as follows: when they're "doing", muscle fibers contract (shorten); when "not doing", they relax (lengthen). To stretch encourages fibers to lengthen—it coaxes them out of any residual voluntary contractions, it persuades them to become flexible and loose. This is one of the relaxation processes on which yoga is constructed—the benefit of asanas (or postures) is largely dependent on the relaxing qualities of stretch.

To demonstrate to yourself how stretch works, all you need do is perform that simple action of dropping your head. After you've let your head hang over your right shoulder for several minutes, or when you feel the muscles on the left side have had enough stretch, then reverse the procedure—hang your head over the left shoulder to distend the right muscles. Move the head back and forth, bob it up and down, and feel how nicely the muscles get stretched. Now drop your head forward, all the way forward as if it were a dead weight, and feel the muscles in back of the neck distend—move the head from side to side, bob it up and down a little—feel the deep stretch down into your back. You may actually experience muscles being pulled right down to the waistline.

75

THE NATURE OF FUNDAMENTAL TENSION

Apparently some individuals are apprehensive about becoming "over-relaxed", as if some tension of the voluntary musculature is required in order to keep the body from falling into a crumpled, unfunctionable heap, like a puppet when its support strings are dropped.

But there need be no such apprehension—the only relaxation we're capable of accomplishing is relaxation of the voluntary (controllable by our conscious or subconscious volition) contractions of the musculature. In addition to voluntary contractions, the human body incorporates a network of fundamental contractions which occur without our voluntary control. These regulate functioning of organ systems such as, for example, the digestive: when food is in the stomach, we cannot stop the stomach and intestines from proceeding with the digestive process, we can only relax voluntary tensions in the stomach area, which tensions may well have been interfering with proper digestion.

Another form of involuntary tension that's present within the musculature is what we call "fundamental tension". Although we strive for optimum relaxation, this natural fundamental tension always remains in any living being's body, even in complete repose. One cannot relax fundamental tension away—it's normal and persists as long as an organism is alive. All we can do by practicing acupressure is relax down to that fundamental tension, or down to "zero repose" as we like to call it.

For a normal person, zero repose is a completely natural state, not something occult, mystic, paranormal, or trance-inducing. It is, to define it very simply, a relaxation of any and all voluntary contractions of the musculature down to the point where only fundamental tension remains. Very young children and animals return to zero automatically between tension episodes.

The existence of fundamental tension has been verified by instrument—electrical impulses were monitored on a sleeping cat and it was found that some small amount of tension remains in muscles even in "complete" relaxation.

It's fundamental tension which makes a living body assume definite postures although it is in zero repose. If you observe a dead animal, you'll note that its limbs and head often fall into positions they would not assume in life, even during deep totally-relaxed sleep.

Fundamental tension also serves to maintain muscles in a state geared for action at an instant's notice. In any living being, the muscles are always on the verge of "doing" even when relaxed. The cat is again a good subject to use in observing the speed with which muscles spring back into action, even from the fullest relaxation. The rapidity with which they revert into "doing" is indeed impressive—to illustrate, just pop a blown-up paper bag a few feet from a sleeping cat. Note how instantaneously every muscle in that cat's body is alert and tensed for action. (Also note the highly annoyed look the cat gives you which asks "Why are you behaving like a dummy?")

We possess the same fundamental tension in our human musculature, and you cannot relax it away, any more than you could relax your stomach away. Therefore, don't restrict yourself in working to relax, just keep letting go as much as possible. On the other hand, don't feel that because you can't get down toward zero repose, the whole thing is hopeless. You don't need to achieve zero in order to benefit from acupressure, whatever degree of relaxation you attain at any stage in your practice will feel enormously beneficial since it means you're burning that much less energy in the form of excessive/unnecessary tension, and those tensions are no longer interfering with the free and full functioning of your system in whatever tasks you may undertake.

ARM AND HAND POINTS

Although it's been my experience that massage of the previously-discussed points at the front and sides of the neck effectively relaxes the entire arms, there are points on the arms and hands to which you may want to apply acupressure. Generally, you can massage any tension-sore points which you locate by feeling for them.

Following are a few specific arm points: there's one just about two inches below the elbow on the upper side of the arm—point E in Fig. 10. Apply pressure here especially for lower arm and hand relaxation, you'll sense the effect in loosening of the hand. About an inch above the elbow on the outside of the arm is another good point (F in Fig. 10). On the upper side of the arm about 2 1/2 inches above the wrist is a third major point (G in Fig. 10). The above three seem always to have point sensation.

We've mentioned head-shaking as an adjunct to acupressure—in a similar vein, there's an oriental method of shaking the fingers and hands which is a direct utilization of vital energy points. The final body points of several meridians are located in the fingertips at either side of the fingernails. When you take hold of a fingernail at its sides and squeeze, you're applying pressure to the points on either side of the nail. In the shaking technique, you take hold of one finger at a time, squeeze gently and shake the finger and hand. This tends to loosen the hand and arm, while pressure on the body points benefits those organ systems influenced by the pertinent meridians.

ACUPRESSURE APPLIED TO THE LEGS

The legs are also an area in which anxiety/tension manifests itself mightily in the human being. At first glance, this may seem somewhat strange because the legs would appear not to be affected by emotions (anxiety/tension) to the extent the eyes, the mouth, the digestive system and such would be affected. But legs are, in fact, acutely and immediately involved in psychological anxiety/tension. The next time you're concentrating intensely —say you're under pressure to complete a crucial and difficult business presentation by a deadline—stop for just a moment and notice how your entire musculature has been brought into play, how fibers throughout your system are tensed to optimum performance levels, and how anxiety over the deadline plays its part in keying up

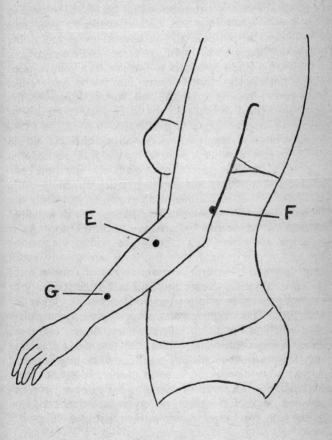

Fig. 10   Arm points

the mechanism. Then notice the legs—note how muscles of the legs and feet are tensed in conjunction with the concentrated intellectual effort on the part of your brain.

When your human system is subjected to any kind of emotional or intellectual stress situation, or to any kind of physical stress, your entire system becomes involved in that stress. When your feet hurt, it shows on your face and in your disposition. If you have a severe toothache, you're not likely to be joyful, pleasant, and eager to join a friend in a tennis match. If you've just seen your beloved pet dog seriously injured by an automobile, your heart may pound rapidly in fright and worry. Whatever the stress—whether mental or physical, whether major or minor—your whole system is affected.

Stresses have repercussions in an exceedingly varied number of ways in many parts of the body. If you undergo a drastic, lengthy, mental stress/anxiety situation, one manifestation of that anxiety may be leg cramping while you're in bed at night. The same symptom, however, can be brought on by pathological conditions such as impaired circulation, which may be causative or contributory. As is true for everything that takes place within the human system, a particular health problem can usually result from any one of several separate causes or from a combination of causes. Years ago, Bill had some tendency of the leg muscles to cramp when he stretched the lower leg and foot. This cramping has since vanished completely as a result of practicing relaxation techniques. However, Fred, a man in his late forties, has severe leg cramping due to impaired circulation resulting from long-standing degenerative disease. Relaxation cannot, of course, cure his cramping. (A word of caution—if you have poor circulation, lack of sensation, or any pathological condition of the legs, don't use massage without first consulting your doctor.)

The human system is a complicated, exquisitely interbalanced mechanism, and numerous different factors can upset the balance of the system. In today's stressful environment, the single factor which most frequently upsets balance is undoubtedly tension. When this happens, balance can easily be restored by simple relaxation. But there are times when the cause of imbalance is of such a nature (being due to tissue degeneration or microbial invasion) that relaxation has only limited, if any, benefits. Our concern in this book is primarily with those myriad occasions where tension is the unbalancing factor. And it is manipulation of vital energy through acupressure which restores balance while simultaneously relaxing tension.

Of the several important vital energy points on the legs, we'll consider first the one located at about the center of the outside thigh, marked H in Fig. 11, a major acupoint in leg relaxation. Tension-soreness in leg muscles will be reflected at this point and pressure applied to it will have truly powerful effects. This particular point is larger in diameter than most others and, while pursuing acupuncture research, I did some experimentation with it on the technique of locating points by touch, based on a slight indentation at the site of the point. More on this in the next section on acupuncture.

As is true for acupressure applied on all other body areas, pressure massage of leg points will relax not only the entire legs but contribute strongly toward relaxation of the human system generally. Along with acupressure, the outer thigh is a good area for some general muscle massage—rubbing, squeezing, pressing, kneading, tapping. Combine this with knuckle pressure on any tension-soreness you may locate, moving your knuckle from spot to spot, applying light pressure each time. When you find a tender vital energy point, work with it a while and let yourself go with the inclination to relax all along the leg and throughout your system.

It's advantageous to devote special attention to point H where massage is particularly therapeutic. When applying pressure to it, use of the knuckle is usually all that's needed although you may find some pressure with the eraser end of a pencil beneficial. Also, pick up the skin surrounding the point between your fingers and squeeze. Use any or all massage techniques, but always keep them so gentle that

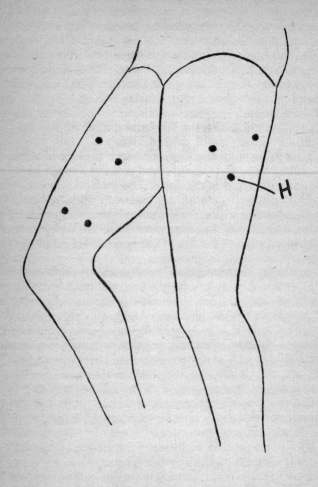

Fig. 11   Upper leg points

relaxation is encouraged—if you exert such vigor that your musculature tenses up against discomfort, you're overdoing it.

There are also some good massage points on the inside of the thigh as indicated in Fig. 11. Again, knuckles and fingers are usually sufficient for applying pressure—use squeezing and other techniques as you feel the need.

Now we move to the lower leg. There's a large group of important points on the outside of the lower leg, as shown in Fig. 12. Using knuckle pressure, you'll probably feel tension-soreness at several of them without difficulty since most of us seem to harbor some degree of chronic tension in our lower legs. One especially valuable point is located toward the front of the leg about seven inches below the knee—point I in Fig. 12. Use a little knuckle pressure on this spot occasionally and see how it helps the lower leg relax. Another major point is located in back of the leg, at the center just where the calf begins—point J in Fig. 12. Rub, squeeze, and apply pressure as needed.

Knuckle pressure and massage on all these lower leg points is enormously useful in foot as well as leg relaxation. It's not necessary to massage the feet per se, because relaxation of feet occurs automatically with overall relaxation of the legs, and particularly with relaxation by point pressure massage of the lower leg. A simple experiment demonstrates how directly lower leg and foot muscles work together. When seated, lift your leg with knee bent. Point your toe. Note how use of calf muscles is required to accomplish the pointing. Bend your foot upwards toward your knee. Note how lower leg muscles participate in accomplishing this action. Since foot muscles work in conjunction with lower leg muscles, relaxation of leg muscles will naturally relax the feet.

On lower leg acupoints, knuckle pressure is excellent and usually sufficient. These points seem to be of the larger variety, and pressure can be centralized adequately by use of the knuckle. However, some pressure with the eraser may be tried if you like.

Should you wish to do some foot massage as an adjunct

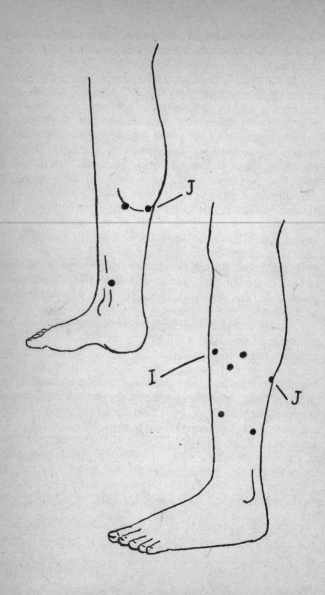

Fig. 12 Lower leg points

to leg treatment, there are, of course, numerous vital energy points located on the feet, just as on every other part of the body surface. Use your hand and fingers to press areas of the feet. If pressure and massage in certain spots is relaxing, use it to aid in your overall relaxation goals.

NO TORSO POINTS USED

When developing this acupressure system, I never used points on the middle or lower torso. The reason is that intuition did not lead me to those points—they weren't zeroed in on as necessary for tension relief. The preferred way to accomplish internal torso relaxation presented itself as being by use of points on the appendages and head, not by manipulating points directly on the torso itself.

Interestingly enough, in acupuncture therapy it's common practice to needle points which are removed from the actual area being treated since the meridians efficiently transport (by means of vital energy) the results of point manipulation along their entire spheres of influence. For this same reason, it's not necessary to massage torso points in order to achieve relaxation of organs and body systems located there.

We do not mean to imply that acupuncture therapists don't use torso points—they are indeed treated and many are remarkably powerful in their effectiveness. But points chosen for treatment on the torso are also usually located some distance from the site of the actual ailment since most schools of acupuncture consider it inadvisable to needle acupoints at the immediate location of illness.

In the practice of acupressure massage, we find torso points somewhat more problematic for a lay person to locate and handle than head, shoulder, arm and leg points. This, combined with the fact that they're not required when the purpose of treatment is simple relaxation, makes use of torso points an unnecessary hassle.

The phenomenal potency with which vital energy transports results of point manipulation is perhaps most dramatically revealed in ear acupuncture. Here is an entire school of practice which utilizes only points on the ear to accomplish successful treatment of ailments throughout the entire body. Better than 200 points have been established on the ear, including a great number which interconnect with all the major meridians. By manipulation of these ear points alone, the same impressive cures can be achieved as by use of vital energy points directly on the traditional meridians. Since utilization of only ear points can accomplish this, it becomes quite understandable why we can achieve such total relaxation throughout the human system by means of acupressure manipulation of just a few face, neck, shoulder and leg points.

RECUPERATION FROM RELAXATION

A curious facet of relaxation is the fact that it sometimes brings about reactions which necessitate a certain amount of recuperation time. This is a facet many people are unaware of; even those who've experienced some of these reactions usually haven't attributed them to the relaxation, believing that they were of some other origin.

We've several times pointed out that relaxation of tension-sore muscles sometimes results in a different kind of soreness. To explain what happens: a muscle that's long been contracted with tension has suffered from lack of movement (or lack of use) just like a muscle that hasn't been exercised (therefore hasn't been used). We think of a muscle that's contracted as a muscle in use. A chronically contracted muscle is in use but it's not being used. After months or years of chronic tension, the muscle suffers from lack of movement just as does the muscle that's been continuously loose and unused for months or years. If a person rarely walks any distance over a period of years, and then suddenly decides to go on a 25-mile hike, his calf muscles will be quite sore the next day. Likewise, a person who has kept most of his shoulder muscles tightly contracted—unused—over a period of years is going to feel soreness in those muscles when they suddenly become relaxed and used. This soreness is sort of like a ramification of tension-soreness. It's similar to how your legs feel after that 25-mile hike. You know the feeling, everyone has experienced it in some muscle area of the body at one time or another. Massaging an unusually tense body point may bring about such soreness in the area. If this develops, refrain from more massage until the point and surrounding muscles have quite recuperated, which usually takes a few days. After the previously-tensed muscles have had a chance to acclimate themselves to their sudden relaxation, to the surprise of finding themselves in use again, they'll feel worlds better. And the more muscles you succeed in coaxing out of chronic contractions, the better you'll feel overall.

A second reaction to relaxation which takes place with some people is overt hurting. This is inclined to occur in the head—the result being headache. A person will say: "When I start relaxing, I get an awful headache. If I stay tense (wound up, keyed up), I'm OK."

The reason this happens is that we use tension/contraction to block pain sensation. Although muscle contraction expresses the pain impulse, additional superimposed contraction can also be used to block that pain impulse. The situation is similar to muscle utilization in the thought process—muscle contraction is required in order for thought to take place, but when a person has something on his mind which is unpleasant or aggravating, he can use tension (additional muscle contraction) to block the thoughts from his conscious mind.

In headache, we can force such strong tension that the pain sensation is blocked. When we reduce that tension a little, the pain, of course, expresses itself. The solution to the problem is continued reduction of tension by which means the pain will itself soon be reduced and finally erased (we are, of course, talking about tension-caused headaches, not those of pathological origin). When tension has been totally resolved, there will no longer be any pain.

Two other reactions which may take place when relaxing an extraordinarily tense area are trembling and jerking.

87

If your eyelids tremble when you relax them, if your lips tremble when you let go of the muscles around the mouth, if your hands tremble or if involuntary jerking (spasm) of the muscles takes place when you relax your arms and hands, that means the amount of tension present is enormous.

Bill had this kind of extreme chronic tension throughout his system when he first began using relaxation techniques. If he simply leaned his head against the back of a chair and let his eyelids go enough so that they'd drop closed, they trembled. This didn't happen when he closed his eyes to sleep at night—the fact is, a person can close his eyes using severely tensed muscles just as most other necessary functions can be accomplished. But when the eye muscles are suddenly relaxed, the unaccustomed loosening causes trembling. The same trembling occurred with his hands when he let his hand and arm muscles go. In addition, his hands also exhibited the reaction which was like an involuntary jerking—that is, the hand muscles would contract and relax involuntarily. These reactions took place for only a short time—as soon as the tension became a bit less extreme, the trembling and jerking stopped.

Bill experienced this same spasm reaction when he relaxed the muscles in the area of his solar plexus (stomach, diaphragm). For years he had walked around with tightly contracted muscles in this area, but despite the duration of the incredible tension, there was only a very short period of jerking when he relaxed.

There's no need to be concerned about trembling or jerking when they take place as a result of practicing relaxation—just take it easy and do only a little at a time, leaving several days between sessions so that the body can accustom itself to its newly relaxed musculature. Within a short time, as your relaxation progresses, the reactions will vanish.

Needless to say, these phenomena can have numerous causes other than tension-relaxation, and if they take place without apparent reason, they should perhaps be looked into medically. However, we know from experience that exceedingly tense muscles will often respond with trembling or jerking when one uses a relaxation method—any relaxation method. This isn't difficult to understand when one considers the vise-like contractions in which tension-fraught muscles are often held. Our experience further indicates that these reactions to relaxation disappear quickly and the only precaution one must take is to go slow and easy so the human system has time to adjust to the relaxation as it occurs. In actuality, very few people will have these responses since such extreme tension is comparatively rare.

TAKE ADVANTAGE OF ACUPRESSURE

We get caught up in the whirlpool of living and taking time out to practice relaxing down to zero repose seems like a waste of time since we're all thoroughly aware of the finite nature of life. Therefore, for most of us, in the beginning, it takes enormous will power to sit and do nothing except relaxation techniques. But after a person has become aware of the improvement in his function and performance, it becomes very much easier to find time for relaxation. Eventually, he becomes so impressed with its benefits that when tensions have built up within him, he automatically makes the time to get relaxed again.

It is our inclination to Do, Do, Do, all the time—we "relax" by playing tennis, or going to a movie, or having a drink in a bar. There is a certain amount of relaxation involved in such things, but every one of those activities can nevertheless be carried on while maintaining tremendous amounts of underlying tension in the body. It is the chronic/excessive underlying tensions that we must oust from our systems and to do this we must practice total, clinical relaxation.

After you've assimilated the techniques and advantages of clinical relaxation, your system will start telling you when it feels too much tension has accumulated and you need a good relaxation session. And as you become more attuned, relaxation will take place much more easily and quickly—so much so that you'll be able to undo the after-tensions of a super-stress episode in your life within a few minutes.

So, take the time to practice letting go. Help your muscles develop the habit of relaxing between actions, coax them out of the habit of remaining tense when not acting. Bear in mind that the stresses and requirements of life will necessitate muscular tensions in order that you can deal with them, and some of those tensions will tend to become chronic or excessive. Don't be discouraged because you have to continue practicing relaxation since the time spent persuading muscles to let go between actions will pay rich dividends in improved performance and increased energy resources. As a result, you'll find yourself leading a richer, fuller, more meaningful life.

The acupressure method described in this book was devised to aid relaxation, and it's fantastically successful in doing so. Acupressure need not be intense, specific, highly trained, occult, or mysterious in any way. As presented in this method, it is simple, gentle, harmless—and as you discover how wonderfully it helps you relax, you'll be eager to take full advantage of its benefits.

There are several methods other than acupressure by means of which we can work toward clinical relaxation. However, of the various procedures available to us which can be practiced independently at home for our own benefit, acupressure massage is by far the most potent and effective. When we stop for a moment to consider that the extension of body point massage—acupuncture, or body point piercing—is a highly developed medical system of proven effectiveness, it's not surprising that point massage itself is a truly powerful therapeutic procedure. None of the other procedures forms a basis for direct cure of disease although each does aid in alleviating ailments since relaxation, no matter how it is accomplished, will always help in relieving conditions which were caused by, or heavily influenced by, tension/anxiety.

It is a simple enough matter to prove to yourself the potency of acupressure—just do it and observe the degree of relaxation which is accomplished. Our own conclusions as to the superior power of acupressure have been drawn from analysis and comparison of the various methods. That is not to say that such as yoga, biofeedback, meditation, syllable concentration, and so on, have little or no value—anything that breaks the tension syndrome to any extent at all has value. Just to sit in your chair (or lie on the floor or on your bed) and focus your attention on consciously letting go of the musculature in one area of your body after another has value. No formal relaxation method has been built around this technique alone, but it is incorporated as part of several methods, including our own (we give a brief description of it in "Preparation for Acupressure", a more detailed description is in our book **Relaxation Renewal**).

Besides its efficacy, here are a few additional advantages which acupressure has over other procedures: 1) you don't need an expensive machine as in biofeedback, 2) you don't need to remove any clothing, or change into exercise clothes, as when preparing to practice the asanas of yoga, and there's no need to learn how to perform stretching postures (asanas), some of which are rather difficult contortions, 3) you don't need to subject yourself to any "secret" theatrics of "initiation" (sometimes at great expense). Although meditation doesn't require equipment, mats, exercise clothes and such, it has the significant disadvantage that it can quite easily be done while maintaining a vast quantity of chronic tension throughout the human body. It does not, of and by itself, bring about relaxation of fixed underlying tensions. What meditation accomplishes is to break the surface tension syndrome, which has a given amount of benefit. But one can only reach complete relaxation in meditation if one is already free of underlying chronic tensions and possesses the facility for letting go. The limitations are clearly recognized by the teachings of yoga—meditation in the form of syllable concentration, for example, forms only a small part of overall yoga training. The asanas are the means whereby underlying tensions within the musculature are relaxed. Another segment of yoga theory makes use of what we call true meditation—that is, meditation where the mind is focused on a beneficial and positive thought, concept, idea or mental image. This, we believe, has strong advantages over syllable concentration because it incor-

93

porates the power of positive autosuggestion. But this is a complex subject in itself which we do not have time to go into at the moment.

Direct manipulation of vital energy flow at body points is the means whereby relaxation is accomplished in acupressure. This same manipulation of energy, while bringing about, concurrently, a balanced energy flow and relaxed mental and physical state, also results in 1) release of waste products from the musculature and other organs, 2) elimination of that pain which is caused by anxieties and tension, and 3) improved functioning of organ systems generally. It is valuable to note that these same advantages occur as a result of vital energy manipulation regardless of whether the method used is acupressure, acupuncture, or moxibustion (heat treatment). Thus, by using simple acupressure, we can gain, to a large extent, essentially the same benefits achieved through more complex manipulations utilizing acupuncture or moxa.

Additionally, acupressure promotes a general state of peaceful well-being. You'll enjoy a calmer outlook on life, and the overall relaxation achieved will result in more beneficial sleep, giving you a feeling of restfulness and adequacy. Being basically relaxed enables you to function to your fullest ability—you perform better in every respect, thus accomplishing more. As a result, your earning power is increased, making possible greater participation in all that life has to offer. These are wonderful benefits indeed to be gained from simply taking advantage of acupressure.

SECTION II

ACUPUNCTURE

ACUPUNCTURE

THE MEDICAL SYSTEM

We include a discussion of acupuncture in this book mainly for the following reasons: 1) a knowledge of acupuncture therapy is most helpful in understanding the reasons behind the efficacy of acupressure massage, and 2) body point massage is and has always been an important alternative to use of needles or moxa in manipulation of body points, and is therefore an integral part of acupuncture therapy.

We have a situation where that homely method of point massage which I'd devised for my own use many years ago solely as an aid to relaxation has turned out to be an ancient, vital component of Chinese medicine. The fact that it is such lends impressive support to our statement that acupressure is indeed a truly effective therapeutic measure. You'll have stronger faith in the technique knowing it's been used for thousands of years, knowing it's related to acupuncture therapy, and knowing the philosophy behind acupuncture itself.

The medical system known as acupuncture therapy is constructed on one principle—the fact that vital energy flows in an organized pattern throughout the human being and may be influenced by manipulation of specific spots on the skin.

All living things (plant and animal) are permeated with this force called vital energy. Throughout the ages, many other names have been given it, one of the more recent being bioplasma, a term employed currently in Soviet research. But since it's always been called vital energy (or vital force, or life force, depending on how you wish to translate the Chinese term) in acupuncture, and we feel this designation is excellent, we've used vital energy throughout our book.

There is no doubt about the existence of vital energy. It's been extensively studied and photographed by means of Kirlian photography, originally in Russia, more recently here in the United States. Such research has provided contemporary scientific "proof" of vital energy; however, its existence was unequivocally accepted by great proto-ancient civilizations on the basis of less technological but equally convincing scientific data.

Vital energy is the life-forming and life-maintaining force diffused throughout all living things. The force is polarized. Its polarities have been designated negative and positive. Chinese terms for the polarities in acupuncture are Yin (negative) and Yang (positive).

When a person is in good health, is relaxed and calm, the vital energy flow is basically balanced. Illness (including illness which is in the making but has not yet overtly manifested itself) will be accompanied by an unbalanced energy flow. The flow can be brought back into balance by manipulation of body points, and this is what acupuncture medical procedure does.

Not only illness, but emotions, thoughts, anxieties, mental effort, physical effort—all affect the vital energy balance. In a living being, this energy oscillates freely—fluctuation from its balance between the polarities does not necessarily indicate a pathological condition. It is when the imbalance becomes excessive and eventually chronic, that it will usually lead to, contribute toward, or be indicative of, a pathological condition.

To illustrate the difference between normal energy fluctuation and pathological imbalance, we'll draw an analogy with hypertension (chronic high blood pressure). If a person runs around the block four times just before entering the doctor's office, or is fraught with anxiety due to fear that he's seriously ill, a blood pressure reading taken immediately will almost certainly indicate high blood pressure. But this reading is the result of physical exertion or mental anxiety and does not necessarily indicate hypertension. Whether hypertension is in fact present must be determined by taking readings when the patient is calm, relaxed and rested from any recent exertion. A high reading under these conditions would probably indicate hypertension. The situation with vital energy is similar. Such things as physical exertion or mental anxiety will cause vital energy flow to deviate from its regular, balanced state. This is normal and does not indicate illness. But a chronic vital energy deviation, a condition where the energy flow remains unbalanced even when the patient is calm and rested would be a strong indication of illness.

In a typical, active person's life, the vital energy doesn't remain always at an even, constant flow since any physical effort (such as manual work or athletics), mental effort (such as intense concentration), or experiencing any kind of emotion will cause the flow to become altered. These are natural deviations. The energy flow should, however, return to balance when the person is completely quiet, relaxed and rested. Living is normally accompanied by polarity changes and predominances taking place in their proper order. There is a series of rhythms, of tensions and relaxations, balancings and unbalancings, predominances of negative or positive energy—all are part of the process of living. When the variation occurs appropriately in accordance with the natural law, there is health. An imbalance which becomes chronic, which no longer behaves properly in accordance with nature, will be the forerunner or reflecter of ill-health.

Since vital energy is the life-force for the entire human system, both mind and body indivisibly, Chinese medicine regards the patient as one "Whole". The mind is not separate, it is an inextricable component of this human system. No part of the human can be treated without involving to some extent all other parts.

Not only does vital energy provide life-force for the human being as an entity, it also functions as the human's link with the cosmos. There is a fundamental energy which permeates the entire universe. Human vital energy is only one manifestation of this fundamental energy, and vital energy retains at all times its relationship with the great fundamental all-controlling cosmic energy. It is for this reason that proto-ancient medicine considered it important that humans function in harmony with cosmic pattern. The human is not isolated from creation, he is part of it.

The human system constantly emits vital energy and must replenish its supply, which is done through breathing ("the breath of life") and through the food we eat and water we drink.

In its diffusion throughout the body, the vital energy moves in an intricate, high-precision pattern of extraordinary complexity. As part of this pattern, it concentrates and channels itself along certain well-defined pathways which strongly influence specific organ systems. These pathways are the meridians. It is by manipulating body points along a specific meridian that the vital energy flow affecting an ailing organ can be adjusted. The manipulation restores vital energy balance which results in healing of illness.

The ability to correct states of illness before they reveal themselves in overt symptoms is one of the most impressive aspects of acupuncture. This is possible because illness manifests itself in disturbed energy balance before outward, noticeable symptoms appear. Such imbalance is determined by reading of the pulses—six on each wrist (see Fig. 13). Organs mirror their functioning in the pulses and an experienced practitioner can determine by means of these pulses which organ systems are off balance (functioning improperly). Acupuncture is then used to restore the proper balance. It is largely due to this method of foreseeing illness that the ancient Chinese doctor was paid as long as he maintained his patient in good health. Payment was discontinued if the patient fell ill, whereupon treatment and medications had to be provided free of charge until the patient again became well.

The process of predicting disease by pulse diagnosis may not seem quite so incredible if we draw another analogy with modern Western medicine. We shall again use the example of hypertension. Much publicity is today

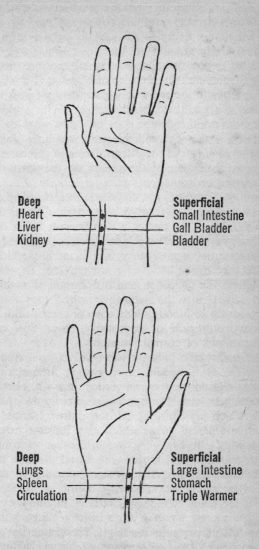

Deep
Heart
Liver
Kidney

Superficial
Small Intestine
Gall Bladder
Bladder

Deep
Lungs
Spleen
Circulation

Superficial
Large Intestine
Stomach
Triple Warmer

Fig. 13   The twelve radial pulses

given to the fact that blood pressure readings are high for many years before the disease reveals itself overtly. People are encouraged to have blood pressure readings taken so that if illness is present, it can be treated before it becomes advanced and obvious.

What is the function of a blood pressure reading? It simply measures the pressure of blood as it flows through the arteries. If the pressure is consistently excessive, overt illness will eventually manifest itself. With a blood pressure reading, the doctor does precisely what the ancient Chinese doctor did with his pulse readings. Just as the sphygmomanometer registers excessive pressure in the arteries, a reading of the pulses on the wrists registers excessive, inadequate, or improper activity of the internal organ systems. Both are diagnostic measures based on the coursing of blood through the arteries. Pulse diagnosis simply carries the matter a step farther, being based on the premise that not only blood pressure but the functioning of internal organ systems is reflected in the blood flow. Since the organs and organ systems are dependent on blood for the collection and distribution of nourishment, it is logical that the manner in which they function in relationship to blood is indicative of their health. If they function erratically or improperly, blood flow could reveal this lack of normal function.

Of the twelve pulses on the wrists, each reflects the condition of a specific organ system. Irregularity in an organ's relationship to the blood flow—a physiological disturbance—would produce irregularity in that blood flow which reveals itself in the pulses. Terms used to describe types of pulses which may indicate trouble are: tight, ropy, slippery, wiry, rough, floating, over-abundant, under-abundant. As is true with blood pressure readings, it is important that the patient be calm, at ease and rested from any recent exertion before a reading of the pulses is taken. Emotions, intense physical or mental effort, anxieties, etc. will affect pulse readings just as they affect blood pressure readings. These transitory factors must be put to rest or removed so that the pulse reading will mirror only the functioning of internal organ systems.

102

BODY POINTS AND MERIDIANS

Although the medical system we are reviewing is called acupuncture (derived from the Latin: acus—needle, and punctura—a pricking), other methods of manipulation besides piercing with needles are used by acupuncture therapists to treat body points. Foremost of these are massage (including pressure) and moxa (heat).

It is not improbable that knowledge of body points and the effectiveness of massaging them preceded discovery of the effectiveness of piercing points. Massage has been practiced since humanity's beginning, and it's certainly logical that some individuals would have noticed that centralizing pressure on certain spots (the vital energy points) is enormously beneficial to health and well-being. When an acupuncture therapist performs massage, he does indeed apply such pressure and it may be that this practice preceded piercing as a medical procedure.

Then too, there are the numerous Western medical professionals who have discovered independently through the centuries that manipulation or treatment of small well-defined skin areas has medical benefits of various kinds for specific types of ailments, or that a diseased condition of an internal organ will mirror itself in manifestations on a certain spot on the skin. A foremost example is what's known in medicine as "Head's zones". Sir Henry Head (1861-1940), a British nerve specialist, noticed that far-removed areas of the skin became hypersensitive to pressure in cases of gall bladder or kidney disease. The painful sensation was on the skin surface and a specific ailment always caused pain at the same place. He categorized the ailments with their corresponding painful skin zones, indicating the diagnostic possibilities, and published his material. "Head's zones" are now included in Western medical training. Doctors have since noted that manipulation of Head's skin zones by heat or massage relieves the pain of kidney or gall bladder attacks. There is no indication that Dr. Head was familiar with acupuncture; nevertheless the skin zones he used are the same as the acupuncture points utilized in treating the same ailments.

Another well-known example of a body point utilized in Western medicine is McBurney's point—a spot on the torso which becomes extremely tender in appendicitis, and is therefore used in diagnosis of this illness.

We might safely assume that throughout the ages, quite a number of professional and non-professional persons discovered the reaction of body points to numerous conditions, including tension. Among those persons, many probably also observed that manipulation of points will alleviate most conditions, including simple tension.

It would seem, then, that knowledge of surface manipulation of points is likely to have preceded knowledge of piercing. Nevertheless, it's traditionally said in Chinese medicine that the principle of acupuncture was first noticed by a warrior who had been struck by an arrow and found that, due to the arrow piercing his skin, a troublesome, chronic pain in a different area of his body had vanished. From this observation, the story goes, was developed the system of piercing body points in order to obtain various medical benefits.

That's the traditional story, but it's also possible that someone, in applying pressure massage with a fingernail or makeshift tool such as a whale bone with a somewhat sharp tip, unintentionally pierced a body point and noticed an enhanced degree of therapeutic benefit from doing so. The practice of piercing points might have come about in more than one way. But whatever the circumstances under which it was discovered, we can be pretty sure it was some type of accidental puncture which revealed the effectiveness of point piercing.

Knowledge of therapeutic body point manipulation was apparently widespread in the proto-ancient world. Only fragmentary remains of this knowledge have survived in most parts of the world—it is solely in the Far East that an entire acupuncture system, with its several techniques, has survived intact to present times. The evidence indicates, however, that during proto-ancient times, many parts of the world practiced some form of acupuncture.

We must pause a moment to explain our use of proto-ancient—proto is taken, of course, from the Greek "protos" meaning "first". The combined term proto-ancient is intended to designate those ancient civilizations which were first in time. Our purpose is to differentiate between what we usually think of as ancient civilizations (Roman, Greek) and those which precede the Greco-Roman by anywhere up to 3,000 years (such as the Egyptian, Sumerian, Mayan, Chinese). What we are in the habit of calling ancient, such as the Greco-Roman, took place approximately 1,600 to 2,800 years ago, whereas previous highly developed civilizations existed as much as 5 and 6 thousand years ago, and some perhaps even earlier. It would seem logical to differentiate between civilizations which were in a state of high developmnt 2,000 years ago and those which were already highly developed 5,000 years ago. The latter we therefore call proto-ancient.

One of the finest medical systems of the proto-ancient world was that of Egypt. The Ebers Papyrus of 1550 B.C., which is among a mere handful of Egyptian medical treatises that have survived to modern times, makes reference to a book on the subject of vessels. No copy of said book has survived, but it's thought to have been about acupuncture. Vessels would have been the meridians—in the Chinese system too, the two central meridians are specifically referred to as vessels: Governor Vessel Meridian and Conception Vessel Meridian. From the nature of the papyrus reference, it is certain that vessels did not refer to arteries, veins or nerves.

The evidence which suggests former widespread knowledge of acupuncture is that various peoples in far-removed parts of the world still practice some type of body point manipulation. Some Eskimos, for example, perform simple acupuncture with sharp stones. An isolated tribe in the Brazilian forest performs acupuncture by shooting minute arrows with blowpipes at specific points on the skin. In South Africa, certain tribes practice scratching of body points to achieve special benefits. Some of these techniques of body point manipulation may have developed independently, some are probably the outgrowth of dissemination of knowledge along trade and travel routes. Proto-ancient civilizations—Mayan, Egyptian, Sumerian, Indo-Chinese, Pre-Incan, etc.—had substantial contact with each other at one time. The concept of a flat Earth was an invention of the Middle Ages—the ancient and proto-ancient world knew full well that it was round. Proto-ancient peoples traveled its circumference regularly. Even its size was measured with a high degree of accuracy— during the ancient Greek period (around 250 B.C.), Eratosthenes of Cyene made the earliest quantitative determination of the Earth's size for which we have records (along with numerous other Earth and Solar System calculations). It's our view that similar calculations for which no records survived were made before the time of Eratosthenes. We cannot probe the matter in great detail here, but one of our reasons is that the calculation systems used were in a state of advanced development when Eratosthenes made his measurements, and such development normally takes place over a lengthy period.

Following the isolation and eventual decline of proto-ancient civilizations, most of their knowledge became dormant, fragmented, or was lost altogether. Centuries and sometimes millennia passed before things known to the ancients were rediscovered, relearned, or redisseminated throughout the world. In our modern era, extensive information on acupuncture has come to the United States only within the past four years. In France and Germany, however, acupuncture therapy has been widely practiced for some time now, while in Russia it's customary procedure for doctors to follow their four-year medical courses with a year's training in acupuncture. It won't be long before knowledge and utilization of acupuncture is once again world-wide.

The current publicity afforded acupuncture in the Western hemisphere may tend to give the impression that Chinese medicine is acupuncture. This is, of course, not the case. Chinese medicine utilizes all therapeutic techniques—including general massage, exercises (breathing and other), surgery, every Western medical technique, and a vast pharmacopoeia of herbal and other natural remedies. Interestingly, the herbal pharmacopoeia is, in many respects, similar to that used by proto-ancient Egypt, which became the system used later by Greece and Rome, then by the Arabic empire, and finally by medieval Europe. When it reached the Middle Ages, the pharmacopoeia consisted of only a few tattered, impoverished remnants of what had once been a complex, efficacious medical system. Nevertheless, these remains formed the nucleus of medical treatment in medieval times. As a matter of interest, just a few of the medicinal herbs and other substances common to the pharmacopoeia of both ancient Egypt and China were: garlic, mugwort, mustard, sesame, liquorice, mint, onion, animal horn, sulphur, potassium nitrate, camphor, pomegranate.

There is a strong tendency today—in the Western World—to condemn herbal and other natural remedies as "nonsense". This attitude disregards the fact that most of our extensively-used laboratory-synthesized medications had their origin in herbal or other natural sources. Aspirin is the prime example, being probably the most widely-used medication among those which originated from natural remedies. The therapeutic substance in aspirin is contained in the bark of the willow tree (salix) which bark was chewed by primitive people to relieve pain. The human being, like all members of the animal kingdom, has a natural instinct that guides him to medicinal plants and other substances when he's ill. Pain led primitive man to eat or chew various plant materials for relief. Willow tree bark was one of them.

This natural instinct is still present in modern man, but is hampered by two factors: 1) the modern conscious mind blocks out instinct as being "unreliable, unscientific," etc., and 2) this particular instinct is, to a large extent, thrown out of kilter by the highly refined foods and laboratory-synthesized medications we consume these days. The instinct was designed to work with foods and medications in their natural form—when the composition of these is greatly altered, by refinement, additives, preservatives and such, the instinct has difficulty coping.

Use of aspirin probably dates back to just about the beginning of mankind, but artificially produced aspirin is a novelty. It was not until the early 19th Century that the pain-relieving substance in willow tree bark was isolated. Following some modification, the substance eventually became a laboratory-synthesized drug manufactured from petroleum-based chemicals. Such is today's aspirin. But you can still chew willow bark and get the same pain-relieving substance—in its natural form.

Another famous medicinal bark from ancient times is Peruvian bark, used to cure malaria centuries before its active ingredient, quinine, was extracted in a laboratory. Then there's our recent plethora of "wonder drugs"—penicillin for example. Proto-ancient Egyptian medicine made extensive use of penicillin in its original form of wheaten-bread mold. Egyptians used other "wonder drugs" too—earth rich in aureomycin was taken for its antibiotic effect in remedying certain illnesses. Our modern laboratories first extracted aureomycin from that very same type of earth. And we all know digitalis is an age-old remedy for heart conditions in its original form as the foxglove plant.

The list of laboratory medicines which originated in nature is very long indeed. True, new medicines have also been synthesized—but the safest, most-used products seem to be those which previously occurred in some natural form, or which have been developed through modifications in the formulation of these originally natural products. Laboratory medicine is essentially an outgrowth and extension of herbal/natural medicine. That one should deny the effectiveness of the other is like a flatworm trying to cut itself in half. If it succeeds, each half will live on its own, but it was one and the same worm to begin with.

Derision is sometimes heaped on many old Egyptian prescriptions because of what seem to be utterly ridiculous ingredients. Some of these ingredients—such as pulverized animal horn—have been analyzed and found to possess medicinal properties. And it is likely that before our modern society rediscovered penicillin and aureomycin, our forbears were properly appalled at Egyptian prescriptions which called for the eating of moldy wheaten bread or aureomycin-rich bits of earth. On the other hand, some other ingredient names in prescriptions may refer to substances entirely different from what the actual word implies. For example, if we were using today certain herbal prescriptions incorporating the following ingredients: cattail, lady's slipper, snowdrops, bluebells, bleeding heart, or babies breath, and a record of these prescriptions was unearthed 4,000 years hence, those future archaeologists, if they accepted those ingredients literally, would understandably be quite perplexed at some of the things we used for medicinal purposes.

But we've digressed too much, let's return to the subject of acupuncture. One of the first questions asked after its introduction into the United States was whether acupuncture itself was bringing about therapeutic results, or whether what occurred was entirely power of suggestion working through the patient's mind. It was proposed that the needles simply served to increase the strength of the suggestion. Several writers even characterized acupuncture as being just another form of faith healing.

Proof that acupuncture therapy does indeed produce therapeutic results of and by itself is very simple: acupuncture is used on animals with immense success. No one can argue that the animal is responding to therapy because of "faith", or because of suggestions that it respond.

Upon accepting the reality that acupuncture itself does produce results, a favorite project undertaken by Western research regarding this ancient art has been to verify the existence of body points by means of one type of electronic instrument or another. It's been subsequently demonstrated with various instruments that acupuncture points coincide with small areas of low electrical resistance—that is, high conductivity—in contrast to lower conductivity of the surrounding area. Electrical potential at body points varies while that of surrounding skin is fairly consistent. Alterations in potential are influenced by the physiological processes of the body and by emotional states.

The total number of points on the human body is enormous. Traditional Chinese acupuncture theory recognizes about a thousand points; however, many more may be located with electronic instruments. By measuring electrophysical skin resistance, one group of scientists located about 400 points on the head alone, every one of them precisely determined.

The system of points on the skin seems to be the body's network of outlets for vital energy, emitting excess or used V-energy just as pores serve as outlets on the skin for perspiration. Since body points are the vital energy contact between internal systems and the outside environment, we can conveniently use these contact points to influence the internal organ systems with which they communicate.

Although V-energy permeates the entire human system, it channels itself rather potently along specific meridians, each of which is a control/reflecter system for the functioning of an internal organ or organ complex. Despite the vast number of points, acupuncture therapy utilizes relatively few, primarily those located on meridians. Figures 14 through 28 show 17th Century Chinese sketches depicting meridians and their points.

There are two central meridians, the first along the center front of the body—called Conception Vessel Meridian, and the second along the center back of the body —called Governor Vessel Meridian. Then there are 12 organ meridians: the Heart, Small Intestine, Bladder, Kidney, Circulation, Three-Heater, Gall Bladder, Liver, Lungs, Large Intestine, Stomach,and Spleen. With the exception of the Governor and Conception Vessel Meridians, all are bilateral.

Meridians do not follow any of the traditional anatomical paths known to Western medicine, and most notably do not coincide with the nervous system. This has been a major argument put forth in denying their existence. However, experimentation with electronic instruments has

110

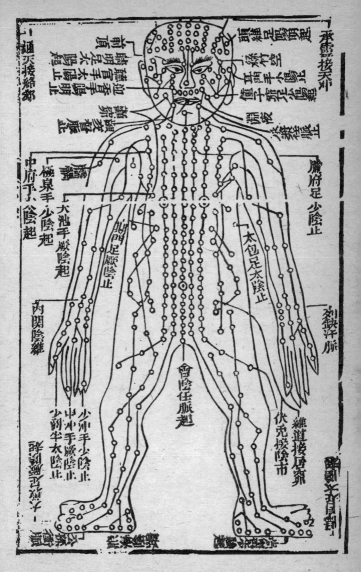

Fig. 14 Comprehensive acupuncture chart—
front of the body

111

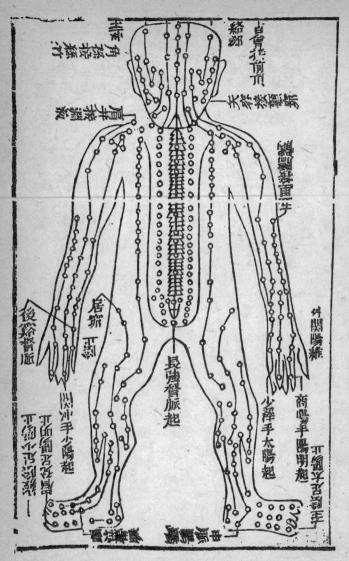

Fig. 15 Comprehensive acupuncture chart—
back of the body

112 、

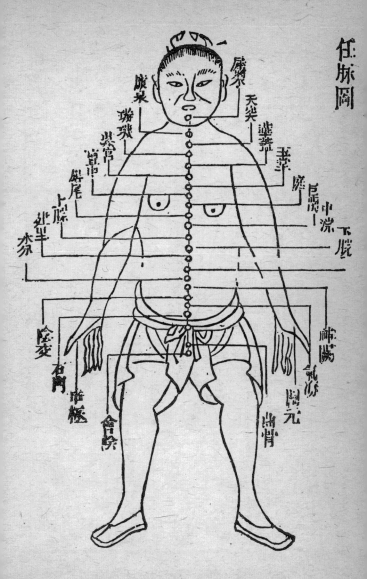

Fig. 16 Conception Vessel Meridian

113

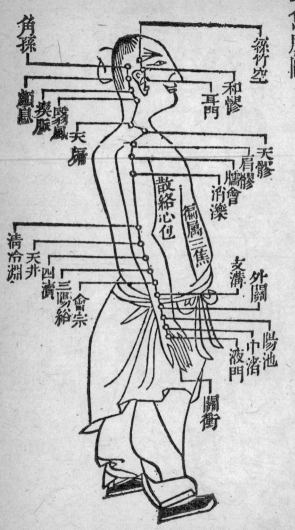

三焦腧圖

角孫
顱息
瘈脈
翳風
天牖
絲竹空
和髎
耳門
天髎
肩髎
臑會
消濼
散絡心包
偏屬三焦
清冷淵
天井
四瀆
三陽絡
會宗
支溝
外關
陽池
中渚
液門
關衝

Fig. 17 Triple Warmer Meridian

114

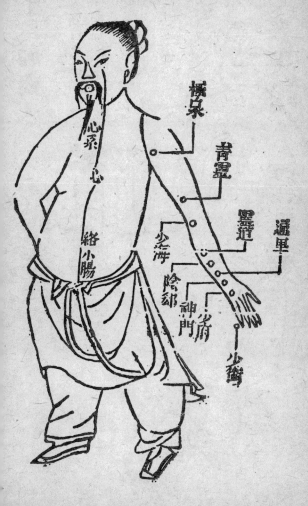

極泉

青靈

靈道

通里

少海

心系

心

絡小腸

陰郄

神門

少府

少衝

陰心經

Fig. 18 Heart Meridian

115

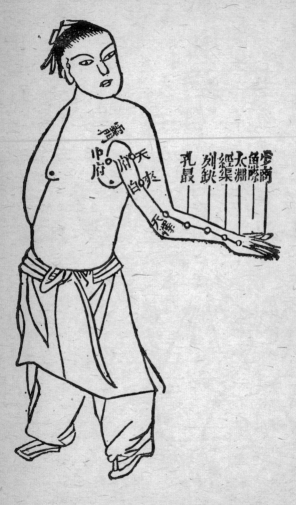

手太陰肺經

中府　雲門

天府　俠白

尺澤　孔最　列缺　經渠　太淵　魚際　少商

Fig. 19　Lung Meridian

116

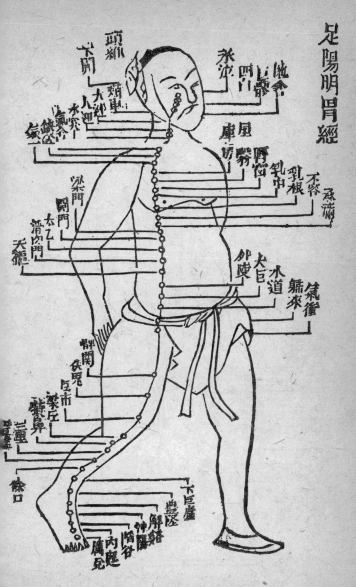

Fig. 20 Stomach Meridian

117

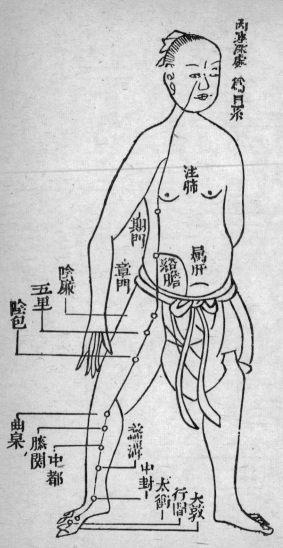

足厥陰肝經

肉凑腠處 屬目系

注肺

期門
章門
陰廉
五里
陰包

屬肝
絡膽

曲泉
膝關
中都

蠡溝

中封
太衝
行間
大敦

Fig. 21 Liver Meridian

118

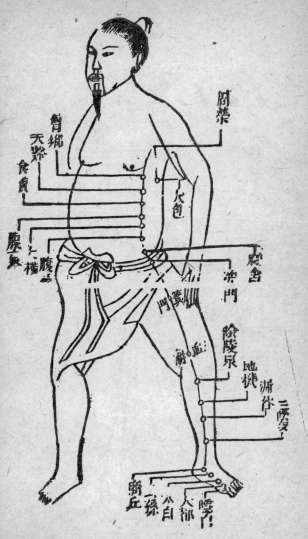

足陰脾經

周榮
胷鄉
天谿
食竇
大包
腹哀
大橫
腹結
府舍
衝門
箕門
血海
陰陵泉
地機
漏谷
三陰交
商丘
隱白
大都
太白
公孫

Fig. 22 Spleen Meridian

119

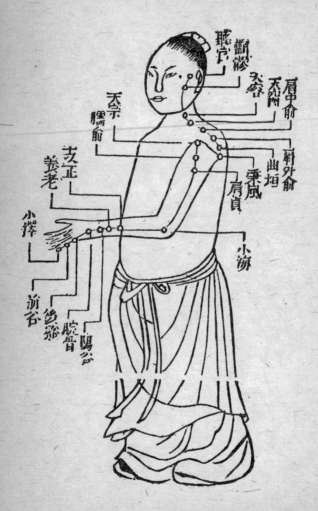

Fig. 23 Small Intestine Meridian

120

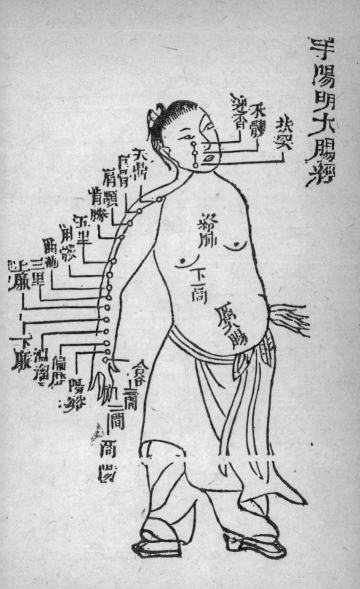

Fig. 24　Large Intestine Meridian

121

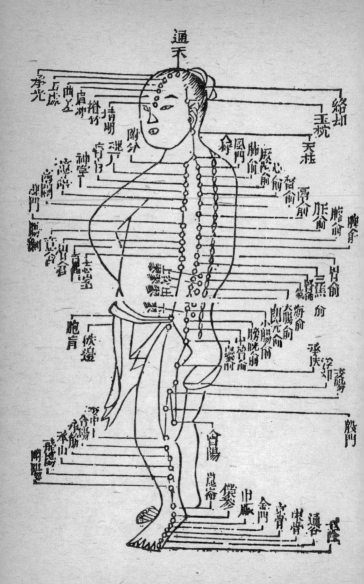

Fig. 25 Bladder Meridian

122

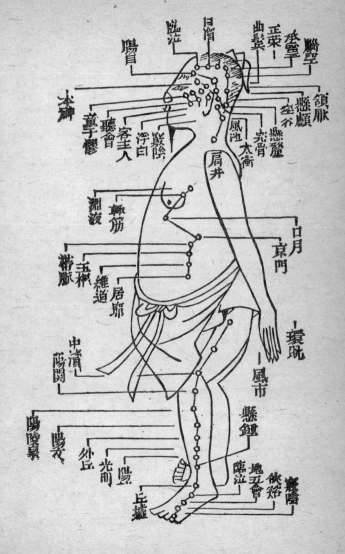

Fig. 26 Gall Bladder Meridian

123

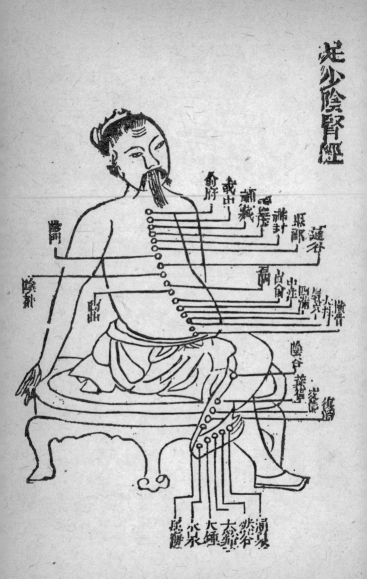

Fig. 27 Kidneys Meridian

124

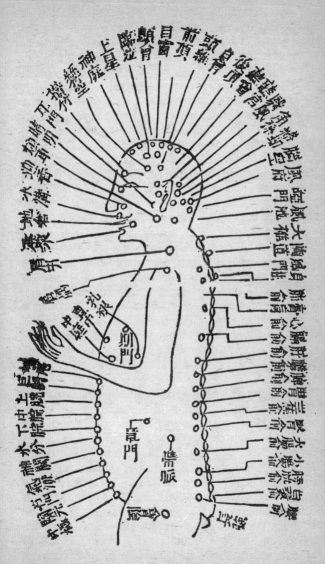

Fig. 28　A composite chart

125

demonstrated the following: if an acupuncture point is stimulated electrically, other points along the same meridian will increase their electrical activity. If the anatomical meridian is cut, electrical stimulation of an acupuncture point on the meridian will not transmit itself to a point beyond the cut. A more commonly-known phenomenon which may be proposed as verification of meridians is that angina pectoris pain follows a path from the heart to the little finger although traditional anatomy cannot explain this link. The path coincides precisely, however, with that of the heart meridian in acupuncture.

Meridians vary extensively in the number of points they possess—for example, the Bladder Meridian has 67, the Heart Meridian only 9. Among schools of acupuncture, there is also sometimes difference of opinion as to whether a certain point belongs on a meridian or not; consequently, body point charts will differ, listing more or fewer points on a meridian. Upon analysis, one soon sees that major points are always the same, only peripheral points are listed in greater or lesser detail, being open to interpretation. Some charts quite simply show just the major points. Additionally, acupuncture charts usually vary in that they show points in somewhat different locations. The reason is that, in practice, actual locations on an individual will vary depending on that particular person's physique. Therefore, exact positions on a chart cannot really be indicated.

In view of the enormous number of points on the body and the fact that the location of a specific point varies slightly depending on the patient's physique, how does a practitioner find the exact point he's looking for? Traditional methods of locating points include 1) measuring distances between points and 2) feeling with the finger for a slight hollow or depression at the site of the point. How are the distances between points measured when there is such diversity of size and build among human beings? By the Acupuncture Unit of Measurement, which is the distance between the ends of the outer folds of the middle phalange of a fully flexed middle finger (right hand for a

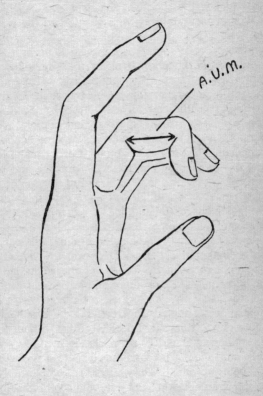

Fig. 29 Acupuncture Unit of Measurement

127

female, left for a male)—Fig. 29. This distance provides a unit of measurement in proportion with an individual's physique. Reminds me of how my Mother used to buy socks for me when I was a child. "Make a fist" she'd say—then she'd wrap the foot of the sock around the fist. If it wrapped comfortably, with a slight overlap for roominess, the sock was the right size. A child's fist is a unit of measurement in proportion to the size of its foot.

Measurement of distances between points is combined with use of the fingers to feel for a slight hollow at the point. With experience, acupuncturists become exceedingly skillful at locating this hollow by touch. As they run their fingers gently over an area of skin, they determine the body point by a slight "give" or "indentation" at its site. Naturally, when I read this in my research on acupuncture, I immediately had to try it. I found it problematic locating points on the face by this method—practice and training would, of course, make it easier. But the point on the outside center of the thigh was quite easy to locate (this is the major outside-thigh point we recommended using in acupressure massage). Sizes of points differ—those on the face are usually small in diameter, whereas this one on the thigh is comparatively large. There was no difficulty zeroing in on this point by feeling for the slight hollow or "give"—I tried it several times and hit it right each time. But I was using my eyes to look at the area where I knew the point was situated, so I couldn't be absolutely sure the fingers had found it. I decided to try without looking, by using fingers alone. To make certain the fingers weren't simply moving on a preconditioned route, I waited several hours before trying. Then, while seated comfortably in an easy chair and looking out the window in the opposite direction, I moved my finger over the outside center of the thigh. When I felt a spot where there seemed to be "give", I pressed and was amazed to find it was the point. To test it, I pressed the area around it, within a half inch to an inch in all directions. No "point sensation" there. Only on that spot where the "hollow" had been felt. Well,

I found this experiment most intriguing, and have tried it several times at widely separated intervals since. Each time, without error, the fingers located the point. Points are generally, of course, by no means this easy for a lay person to locate by the touch method. Both the fact that this particular point is rather large, and the fact that point sensation may be felt here when you press so you know you're on the right spot, serve to make this one comparatively easy to find by touch.

Today's acupuncturists have electronic instruments available to them for locating points. Many of these were developed from devices mentioned earlier which were invented for purposes of proving electrically that points actually exist. Recently, Soviet scientists developed the Tobiscope, a point-locating apparatus which incorporates knowledge gained from their research on bioplasma through use of Kirlian photography. Instruments are presently being designed which will monitor vital energy flow in the meridians, thereby simplifying, in many cases, both diagnosis and treatment by acupuncture.

Although the system of acupuncture commonly practiced today utilizes points on the entire body, modern practitioners in the People's Republic of China have also revived ear acupuncture, an equally ancient therapy method. The more than 200 ear points, being connected directly or indirectly with all meridians, can be utilized to affect vital energy in the same manner that points on the meridians themselves are used. Treatment by manipulating (needling, moxibustion, massage) ear points was common during ancient times in China and continued to be practiced in rural areas as folk medicine right through the numerous vicissitudes of various political and medical establishments. Currently, ear acupuncture has been moved into the realm of serious research, has been employed successfully in treating numerous ailments, and offers tremendous potential for present use and additional future development.

METHODS OF TREATING BODY POINTS

The three basic methods by which vital energy points are manipulated or treated are:

1. Piercing with needles.
2. Applying heat with moxibustion.
3. Massaging with the fingers or a massage implement.

PIERCING WITH NEEDLES. The first method involves insertion of needles into vital energy points. Needles are made of various materials depending on availability and preference of individual acupuncturists or schools of practice. Some practitioners believe the choice of material is of great importance, others feel it is unimportant or of relatively little importance. Many feel that the puncture itself is the only therapeutic factor. It is indeed scientifically accepted that puncture—whether done by fish bone, thorn, wood splinter, or metal needle—works to reestablish vital energy equilibrium. The differences of opinion are on whether the degree of effectiveness achieved by puncturing will change with various materials, or whether the material is itself of no significance.

It is agreed, however, that shape, diameter, and length of the needle do affect the degree of vital energy manipulation, and these factors are considered in choosing the proper needle for a specific treatment. Numerous techniques are used to achieve the most advantageous effect of needling in given circumstances—techniques include length of time inserted, depth of insertion, warming of the needle, twirling the needle, vibrating it, or pushing it up and down. Needles are usually inserted into the skin only to the depth of a few millimeters.

Insertion of the needle precisely in the acupuncture point is of overriding importance, both in order to accomplish the desired treatment results and to avoid injury or other adverse effects. Misplaced insertion may cause severe pain, loss of consciousness, vomiting, etc. A needle skillfully and correctly inserted in the point is painless or nearly so.

The degree of effect a therapist achieves with the needle may be controlled (decreased or increased) in the following ways: 1) by the thickness of the needle—a thicker needle produces more effect, 2) by manipulation of the needle—twirling, pushing it up and down, vibration, etc., produce more effect, and 3) by depth of insertion—deeper insertion produces more effect. Needles may also be manipulated by means of electrical stimulation, by being hooked up to an electronic device which causes them to pulsate rapidly. This is used primarily in operating-room analgesia where needles must be manipulated continuously over long periods of time. In disease treatment, manual manipulation is preferred because it can be better controlled and varied in accordance with the requirements of the individual patient's condition.

Most acupuncture needles used today are of stainless steel, silver or gold. Use of gold is currently rather popular in certain parts of the world although many acupuncturists say the only advantage of gold (or silver) needles is that they impress the patient. Gold has the possible disadvantage that it's rather soft and may bend if it should hit a bone, making extraction of the needle slightly difficult.

No medication is used on needles in traditional acupuncture. The therapeutic result is from the action of the needle alone.

Specific points or combinations of points are treated for specific ailments. The number of points needled varies considerably depending on the illness and on the individual patient's degree of response to acupuncture. Sometimes a single needle suffices, at other times fifteen or more points may be needled. Points treated are often far removed from where the illness is centralized. Acupuncture theory generally recommends treating points located at a distance from the actual site of illness, and at times, on the opposite side of the body. Points treated are, however, on the meridian linked with the ailing organ. Since vital energy is effectively influenced at numerous points along the meridian (on both sides of the body), it is usually unnecessary and unwise to treat the actual site of illness where pain, inflammation, swelling, etc., may be present.

APPLYING HEAT WITH MOXIBUSTION. Moxa, the second method of treatment, is the burning of dried mugwort leaf (Artemisia) on the acupuncture point. Moxa is an anglicization of the Japanese "mo ku su" meaning "burning herb". A small cone of mugwort is placed on the body point and lighted at its top. An incense stick is used for lighting, never a match. The herb is permitted to burn down until the heat becomes uncomfortable, it is then removed before an actual burn with possible scarring can occur. Moxibustion is a much-used home remedy in the Far East since a patient who's learned which points to treat and how to use the mugwort can follow through on his own treatment.

Another way to use moxa is in stick form—a cigarette-like stick of mugwort is ignited and held close to the acu-point until the skin becomes uncomfortable. It's then removed, to be returned when the body point has cooled. This is done several times in a treatment session.

Sometimes a small cone of moxa is burned at the top of an acupuncture needle, in which case the needle acts as conductor of heat. This is particularly effective in relief of muscular pain as well as pain referred from internal organs.

MASSAGING WITH THE FINGERS OR A MASSAGE IMPLEMENT. The third method of point treatment—massage—is often used by acupuncture therapists in preference to needles when treating children, the aged, or the extremely debilitated. Manipulation of points by needles engenders too strong an effect for persons in those groups. Therapeutic massage of the proper body points by an acupuncturist can bring about essentially the same medical benefits as needling, but on a substantially milder scale. As is the case with all Oriental techniques of body point manipulation, remedial massage of acupuncture points is intended to restore the vital energy balance. Pressure, friction, movement, and percussion are used.

132

Pressure. Pressure is applied by means of a special implement, by a fingernail, or by pressing with fingers or knuckles. The traditional implement is in the form of a rod with a rounded or ball-tipped end. That part of the implement which comes in contact with the skin is of an electrically non-conducting material such as plastic, wood, bone, etc. A fingernail may be used in somewhat the same way as the implement, the nail being of a horny non-conducting material. If you press a point using a fingernail, the sharpness of the nail effectively localizes pressure.

Probably the most frequently-employed means of applying pressure is simply pressing with fingers or knuckles.

Friction. If the fingernail is sufficiently long so that the practitioner's finger itself does not touch the patient's skin, the fingernail may be used to scratch a point for the purpose of building up a slight static charge which will discharge itself upon reaching a certain level. A minute charge, it is nonetheless capable of substantial penetration along the meridian. The scratching, or friction, should be light and must be done in only one direction. A non-conducting massage instrument may be used to build up a slight charge in the same manner.

A second form of friction is deep friction massage. This involves applying pressure to the point with a finger or knuckle, then moving the upper layers of skin back and forth rapidly so as to apply friction to underlying surfaces.

Movement. The movement techniques of rubbing, squeezing, and kneading are done with the fingers. These are quite the same as described in acupressure massage.

Percussion. Using fingers or knuckles to strike the body points is also done in essentially the same manner as described in acupressure massage. Acupuncture therapists generally strike from a distance of 2 to 4 inches and hit one point no more than three times in one session. The elbow or heal of the hand are also used for percussion.

CHOICE OF MASSAGE TECHNIQUE is a matter of the practitioner's preference. All techniques are effective.

Massage used by acupuncturists is basically the same as

the acupressure method we developed independently. This is not surprising in view of the fact that massage techniques are instinctive; those of diverse eras and diverse civilizations have been fundamentally alike.

CONDITIONS TREATABLE BY ACUPUNCTURE

All illness is accompanied by imbalance in functioning of the human system. Often, imbalance is itself the cause of illness, as when brought about by severe tension/anxiety/stress over a long period of time. In the case of infectious diseases, the imbalance is due to damage resulting from microbial, viral, or fungal invasion. Or imbalance may be the result of tissue degeneration, as in cancer. Sometimes imbalance results from a combination of detrimental factors which serve to undermine the normal functioning of the human system.

Acupuncture treats illness by restoring balance. This is accomplished by balancing the vital energy flow which influences and reflects the condition of all physical and mental human processes.

An enormous number of ailments are treatable by acupuncture. Generally speaking, acupuncture may be effective in curing all ailments with the exception of those resulting from invasion by infectious organisms, and those of a degenerative nature such as cancer. In the latter two categories, acupuncture is unable to restore balanced functioning, being capable only of symptomatic relief.

Acupuncture doesn't always work, even with illnesses where the rate of cure is extraordinarily high. The duration of the disease, how much damage has been done, and the general state of the patient's constitution are among the factors which will influence the effectiveness of acupuncture therapy. A patient may also have several ailments concurrently, not all of which are treatable by acupuncture. Still, in the case of treatable diseases which have progressed so far as to be beyond a cure by acupuncture, it is sometimes possible to arrest the condition so it doesn't become worse, or a severely incapacitating condition may sometimes be sufficiently relieved through acupuncture to make possible the resumption of a reasonably normal life.

There is no method of treating disease which is 100% effective at all times. On the other hand, most methods will produce good results from time to time. The criterion by which a method must be judged is: how consistently does it succeed with a relatively high level of effectiveness and cure. Acupuncture, over thousands of years, has demonstrated its ability to produce impressively consistent cures and improvements.

It must always be remembered, however, that many diseases, such as those caused by infectious organisms, are curable by other medical systems whereas acupuncture is of little or no value. Among certain individuals, there is some tendency today to claim that acupuncture is the supreme form of medical treatment, other forms being inferior and used only by doctors who are not fortunate enough to belong to that elite corps which makes a patient well by magically adjusting his vital energy instead of doping him with drugs, carving him in surgery, or such other lesser methods. This is a mistaken attitude.

Individuals who claim a supreme status for acupuncture sometimes designate as superior those proto-ancient medical establishments which used vital energy manipulation. Several—including the Egyptian, Chinese, and Aztec—did concern themselves with that vital force, the interplay of which regulates/reflects all processes of the body. They aimed to influence that force in order to reestablish equilibrium in processes which were off-balance. But they were equally concerned with other means of treating human ailments, including herbal medicine (the counterpart of today's drugs) and power of positive suggestion (psychosomatic medicine). Surgery was also highly developed and used when indicated.

In the Western world, the only medical system which survived with any degree of intactness into Roman and Medieval times following the decline of proto-ancient civilizations was the system based on herbs and other natural material substances. The reason it survived rather than one of the others, such as acupuncture, was mainly a matter of chance. In China, both acupuncture and knowledge of herbs survived as folk medicine throughout several upheavals in their civilization. But after the decline of Egypt, knowledge of vital energy was totally lost to the Western world, which turned to the more material herbal medicine. A knowledge of herbs and their therapeutic qualities may be acquired, applied, and passed on to following generations perhaps more easily than a knowledge of body points and vital energy or the role of suggestion in medicine. Also, herbs were real, tangible, and most were available free for the picking in any open field. Our modern Western medical system, based on chemicals (drugs), grew out of these herbal remedies, and some of us are inclined to believe that it—being "real" and "tangible"—is the supreme system, others being of only passing interest, as curiosities, sort of. We are no more correct in our assessment than are the aforementioned acupuncture zealots.

It is a mistake to discard or denigrate any system which has demonstrable usefulness. All medical practices which have proved they can help us must be fully utilized to the best of our ability.

A sampling of ailments which may be cured or alleviated by acupuncture follows. This list does not, by any means, include all treatable ailments, and an ailment may not respond in all cases.

Nervous System, Psychiatric: depression, anxiety, timidity, fear, insomnia, nervousness, temper tantrums, irritability, obsessions, nervous trembling, dizziness, hysterical paralysis.

Head: headaches, head congestion, neuralgia, migraine, tics.

Respiratory: hay fever, asthma, sinusitis, laryngitis, bronchitis.

Cardiovascular System: angina, palpitations, fainting, cardiac insufficiency, high or low blood pressure, phlebitis, hemorrhoids.

Musculature, Osteal System: rheumatism, sciatica, lumbago, slipped disc, cramps, frozen shoulder, rheumatoid or osteoarthritis.

Sexual: impotence, frigidity, sterility, menstrual pain and abnormal flow, hot flashes, excessive sexual desire, lack of sexual desire.

Gastrointestinal: ulcer, colitis, indigestion, constipation, diarrhea, nausea and vomiting, heartburn, rectal prolapse, cramps.

Urinary: bed-wetting, cystitis, lack of bladder control, renal insufficiency.

Skin: sweating problems, itching, acne, eczema.

General: fatigue, anemia, pain, weakness during recuperation from disease or an operation, lethargy.

The number of treatments necessary to bring about a cure by acupuncture varies considerably. There is also extensive variation in type and speed of response to acupuncture therapy. Some patients improve immediately upon insertion and manipulation of the needles whereas others show little improvement until after several treatments. An individual patient's response to a single treatment may be noticed during the treatment or several hours or days later. With most people, the response is of a positive nature engendering continuous betterment of the patient's condition; however, in a few cases the condition will become somewhat worse before it becomes better (which also occurs in the practice of other medical systems).

PAIN RELIEF

Acupuncture may be used to relieve pain, although simple removal of symptoms without curing the underlying condition is discouraged by traditional schools. Symptoms are nature's warning system and one must take care not to remove the warnings without correcting the problem.

However, in advanced irreversible conditions (such as chronic osteoarthritis) acupuncture is used for symptomatic relief, particularly pain. Since these are advanced conditions in which the source of pain cannot be cor-

137

rected, the pain will, of course, eventually return, just as it returns when the effect of any other form of pain relief (drugs such as aspirin, morphine) has worn off.

Suggestion no doubt plays a part in acupuncture pain relief just as it does in all other methods of easing pain. The effectiveness of an analgesic drug is usually enhanced by the power of suggestion. Also, it is well known that a placebo—a pill containing no medically active ingredients at all—when given to patients who believe they are getting a pain-killing drug, will effectively relieve pain in 14 to 33 percent of those patients.

ACUPUNCTURE ANESTHESIA/ANALGESIA

The insertion of needles in certain points and the continuous manipulation of those needles will produce anesthesia in a large number of patients. Actually, a more accurate term for the condition produced by acupuncture is analgesia. Anesthesia means a loss of all feeling—including pain, touch, heat, cold—either locally or totally depending on how it's given. But, when a patient is prepared for an operation by acupuncture, there is no loss of feeling, there is only removal of pain sensation. The patient still feels everything that's going on—the scalpel cutting, the surgeon handling organs—but there is no pain. Therefore the effect is, in reality, one of analgesia.

The points used in achieving acupuncture analgesia are determined by the operation which is to be performed. It is continuous manipulation of the needles in these points which produces continuing analgesia. Originally, this manipulation was accomplished by manually twirling the needles. But uninterrupted action was essential and many hands were required to twirl the necessary number of needles, first in preparation for the operation, then during the entire length of the operation. Since this was quite tiring for the therapists, an electrical stimulator came into use and the needles are now hooked up to this instrument which provides up to 200 pulsations per second.

Not all people can be adequately analgesized by acupuncture to permit having surgery performed. Patients must be tested beforehand to determine whether sufficiently deep analgesia can be achieved. Generally, those who respond strongly to ordinary acupuncture treatment will be most likely to achieve analgesia by this method.

POWER OF SUGGESTION IN MEDICINE

As has been the case with many facets of acupuncture therapy, acupuncture analgesia has been described by some Western medical people as just another application of suggestion or autosuggestion. The contention is that results are achieved wholly by suggestion, the needles serving as little more than dramatic props. Again this is easily refuted by the fact that animals are effectively analgesized by acupuncture. It is certain the animal doesn't lose its sense of pain because of suggestion or because it's impressed by the drama of needles piercing its skin.

Due to the nature of the human mind, suggestion no doubt often plays a role in human acupuncture analgesia, since suggestion contributes to just about every medical action performed by or to the human being. If suggestion succeeds in enhancing the degree of analgesia, this would seem a highly desirable situation rather than something to be discarded as unacceptable. There are on record cases where patients achieved analgesia during the entire period of an operation solely through use of autosuggestion. Such achievements should be applauded and encouraged rather than contemptuously rejected. Whether analgesia is accomplished by means of acupuncture, autosuggestion, or a combination of the two, such analgesia has the distinct advantage of not exposing a patient to the many possible deleterious effects of chemical gas or drug anesthesia.

The fact is that suggestion plays a strong part in most any kind of medical procedure—regardless of the medical system being used, how strong a part being dependent mainly on the suggestibility of the individual patient rather than on the type of medicine practiced. The term "suggestion", as used in Western medical writings, tends to come across as something not quite legitimate, something phony perhaps, which produces only imaginary instead of genuinely health-giving results. We do not agree with this —suggestion is very real, and produces genuine results. Whether they are health-giving depends on what words were used in the suggestion and the attitude of the person making the suggestion. Positive, beneficial suggestions often produce better, more genuinely health-giving results than do chemical drugs. There is always a certain amount of risk involved in use of medicinal drugs, yet their value is fully recognized and we certainly acknowledge that value. But we feel the value of suggestion should also be recognized. Both have their potential benefits, both have their shortcomings. Both should be used for the benefit of humanity to the utmost degree possible.

In medicine, the ideal approach is recognition of the potential power of suggestion concomitant to use of any and all methods of treatment, whether drugs, herbs, acupuncture, or whatever.

But despite the overall power of suggestion, an interestingly significant number of patients are not strongly affected by a doctor's words/attitudes. Affluent persons in this category will see several doctors for an opinion on a condition, weigh the various opinions and make their own decisions. I read recently of a major sports figure who follows this procedure every time he suffers an injury.

In truth, none of us is totally helpless in a world replete with suggestions being constantly hurled at us. We have particularly strong defenses against detrimental suggestions. To what extent an individual accepts or rejects a suggestion depends on his innate personality makeup, his education, his experience, the source of the suggestion, and the circumstances surrounding the suggestion. Nevertheless, it is safe to say that the majority of human beings will usually be influenced by the suggestions of a doctor, whether those suggestions are in the form of words, attitudes, or actions.

Kirlian photography and other vital energy research has clearly demonstrated the powerful effect suggestion, whether autosuggestion or suggestion from other persons, can have on a human's vital energy system. Knowing this, it's not difficult to comprehend how it is that beneficial suggestion can genuinely help restore health, at times more easily and effectively than drugs. Negative suggestions, on the other hand, can be truly detrimental, making restoration of health more problematic or even impossible.

It's not unlikely that in some acupuncture cases, the cures are actually the result of positive suggestion. It's also not unlikely that some patients cured after a visit to a Western doctor are cured by the favorable suggestion of having make the visit, purchased the prescription, and swallowed the drug, and not actually by the action of the drug. In both cases, the positive suggestion that something was being done for him which would help him get well encouraged the patient to rally his body's natural disease-fighting forces and overcome his ailment.

However, it's as unwise to look upon suggestion—or, in its expanded form, the power of "self-healing"—as a supreme and total medical system, discarding all others, as it is to do so with any other medical system. Suggestion (or self-healing) has its definite limitations as do all forms of medical therapy. No beneficial medical system should be discarded, all should be used to the best of our human ability.

SECTION III

RELAXATION PROOF

RELAXATION PROOF

THE REASON WHY AND HOW ACUPUNCTURE WORKS

There is, and has always been, a good deal of questioning as to why and how acupuncture works.

The textbooks state that acupuncture accomplishes four things: 1) it sedates, 2) it stimulates, 3) it relaxes, and 4) it alters physiological function by reestablishing balance between the two energy polarities. They state that how acupuncture accomplishes these things is not known—"no one knows how or why acupuncture works".

On the other hand, we state that what acupuncture does is to relax, and that sedation, stimulation, and altered physiological function are concomitant results of this relaxation. Relaxation can sedate. Relaxation can stimulate. Relaxation will reestablish vital energy balance. How acupuncture accomplishes these things is by relaxation.

Instead of relaxation being one of several results of acupuncture, it is the single common denominator by means of which all other results are achieved. Manipulation of vital energy points brings about relaxation. And the method of manipulation which is the most potent relaxant is puncture with needles.

It is our opinion that the major part of acupuncture's therapeutic benefit is due to the extraordinarily high degree of relaxation induced by puncture of vital energy points. The resultant relaxation of organs and their support systems encourages them to function fully and normally. In this way, the cure of numerous ailments is achieved.

We think that relaxation may not be the total 100% explanation for why and how acupuncture works, but it plays a far more important role in the therapeutic benefits than has previously been recognized, being responsible for perhaps 90% of what acupuncture achieves. The factor responsible for the remaining 10% most likely involves the nature and behavior of vital energy, a substance about which we know very little at present.

Let us consider briefly the traditionally indicated functions of acupuncture, placing them in relationship to relaxation:

ACUPUNCTURE SEDATES. Where use of sedation is indicated, acupuncture may perform this function in place of drugs. It is also true that practicing any relaxation method, such as certain forms of yoga or meditation, will sedate if sedation is needed.

ACUPUNCTURE STIMULATES. When energy or tone are below par, acupuncture often engenders a remarkable new vitality. It is also true that in the case of persons whose energy and/or organ tone are poor due to tension/anxiety, relaxation, by whatever means it is accomplished, will bring about an apparently amazing increase in vitality and improvement in tone.

ACUPUNCTURE RELAXES. Acupuncture therapists have said that correcting the overactivity or underactivity of organs results in relaxation. We say the opposite—it is the relaxation which results in correction of the over-activity or underactivity of organs. For example, if your stomach is relaxed, it will produce the proper amount of required digestive juices to perform its work (assuming it is organically normal). If it is tormented by extreme anxiety/tension (in reflection of an intense stress situation in which you, as a person, find yourself), its production of juices and performance of the digestive process will go awry. It is not brought back to proper functioning by directly decreasing or increasing the amount of juices produced or changing the way the stomach wall is doing its job. It's brought back to proper functioning by relaxing, which automatically returns the juices and stomach wall

146

to their correct workings. (A medication can alter a specific digestive action—by coating the stomach wall, for example—but this is temporary, symptomatic relief; it does not, in itself, return the stomach to normal functioning.)

ACUPUNCTURE MODIFIES PHYSIOLOGICAL FUNCTIONING. Acupuncture theory states that by reestablishing balance in the vital energy flow, it can correct mental depression or excitation; remedy insomnia, constipation, menstrual problems, impotence, etc. We state that such conditions as these are usually caused by, or strongly influenced by, anxiety/tension, that relaxation reestablishes balance, and that any relaxation technique practiced by the patient, or by a practitioner on the patient, would be likely to improve such disorders. The difference is that acupuncture is by far the most potent relaxant and thus effects much greater improvement and usually a cure. When normal body systems are relaxed, they function well.

We present our case as follows:

ACUPUNCTURE REESTABLISHES BALANCE.

RELAXATION REESTABLISHES BALANCE.

Acupuncture, which is manipulation of the body points —whether by needle, moxa, or massage—relaxes (balances) the energy flow which relaxes (balances) the functioning of the organ systems affected by the particular points. We do not think of puncturing skin with a needle as a relaxant, but heat (moxa) and massage, two well-known means of relieving tension, are also commonly used to treat vital energy points.

HEAT RELAXES—heat applied by means of burning moxa is a major part of acupuncture treatment. In manipulation of body points by heat it is quite easy to comprehend that therapeutic results are probably due largely to relaxation.

MASSAGE RELAXES—massage manipulation of body points is usually the only acupoint therapy used on children, extremely debilitated, or very elderly persons. Because the effect of needles is too powerful, massage is used in their place when treating these groups. If simple massage can accomplish, to a great extent, the same results as needle piercing, then it is not illogical that relaxation is a major part of how acupuncture works. Piercing a body point has a certain occult-like mystery about it which gives the impression the entire procedure is eerie and in-comprehensible, but there's nothing occult, eerie or mysterious about massaging a body point. If we take note that point massage can accomplish to a large degree the same medical benefits as piercing a point, the piercing tends to lose a lot of its eerieness and become a more down-to-earth, factual phenomenon. We could state the comparison in this manner:

• Massage relaxes (does away with tension), and massaging specific body points can result in a specific medical benefit.

• Piercing the same body points can result in the same medical benefit, and it is therefore likely that a major part of the result achieved by piercing is also due to relaxation, just as in use of massage.

When you perform pressure massage on vital energy points, using your fingernail to centralize pressure on a tense, sensitive point has a most relaxing effect. Much the same effect is achieved by using a pressure implement—a slender paint brush handle, the rubber eraser on the end of a pencil, or an implement manufactured specifically for the purpose of massage. You can easily feel the relaxation reaction when applying precision pressure on a tense point by use of an implement or fingernail.

It is only a small step further from such an implement or fingernail to a needle which actually punctures the point. (If you press hard enough, you will, in fact, puncture the point with your fingernail.) It is certainly logical that the relaxation benefit achieved with the implement is also present when that implement is made pointed and punctures the body point.

Some actions performed with a needle, such as vibration, can also be performed with a fingernail. If you apply gentle pressure and move the nail back and forth rapidly (not over any distance, just vibrate it) on the vital energy point, you'll feel an enhanced relaxation benefit. But you must use a body point which presents tension soreness so you can feel the relaxation taking place; if you use a point not affected by tension, there will be no relaxation since the areas influenced by the point are already relaxed. (If you experiment with this action, we repeat—do not perform any action so intensely as to pierce the acupoint. Piercing must be done only by professionals trained in acupuncture.)

Vibration is frequently used in needle acupuncture. When you try it on the body point surface using your fingernail and observe the result, it's easy to see that vibration does produce enhanced effectiveness and it logically follows that vibration would also increase the effectiveness of puncture by a needle. Analgesia, perhaps the most dramatic and intriguing application of acupuncture, is achieved by hooking up the needles to electrical instruments which provide perpetual vibration (or pulsation).

MANIPULATION IS THE DETERMINING FACTOR. It is the manner of manipulation rather than the type of object used for acupuncture which determines the degree of response. Acupuncture theory generally concedes that the object employed to make the puncture is of little or no importance—it could be a needle, fish bone, thorn, or any other such thing. It is the puncture itself and manner of puncture which produce the results. However, the object's diameter, the length and depth of insertion, heating the object, or moving it (twirling, vibrating) will influence degree of response and acupuncture results. This is again analagous to massage—it is the manipulation of the acupoints that brings results. The sharp puncture tool is essentially another manipulation implement, just as the fingers are massage manipulation implements. The great difference is that puncture manipulation usually produces far more effect than massage manipulation. Thus an effectiveness scale might read:

149

Low: Massage
High: Simple puncture
Higher: Certain manipulations performed with the object used for puncturing.

Since the same results can be achieved with these three means of point treatment, the only variation being in the degree of result, it is logical that there's a common underlying something which takes place to bring about the results. We believe this something is relaxation, and that this is the why and wherefore that makes acupuncture work.

THE VITAL ENERGY SYSTEM

Although the vital energy network is a system in its own right and not synonomous with the nervous system, musculature, or any other traditionally acknowledged anatomical system, it does nevertheless exert simultaneous effects on both the nervous system and musculature when the vital energy is influenced in any way. Thus, application of pressure to a point affects not only vital energy flow, but simultaneously affects the nervous system and musculature. In actuality, the entire human system is affected, to a greater or lesser degree, by that application of pressure to one vital energy point since this energy is diffused throughout the body. But we shall specifically consider the nervous system and musculature at this time.

In the first place, anything that produces sensation in the human system must involve the nervous system. Body point sensation and tension sensation therefore involve the nervous system. Furthermore, manipulation in any way of any body function will cause reaction in, and involve, the nervous system. (But since the vital energy system does not anatomically coincide with the nervous system, body point behavior cannot be explained away as merely a facet of the nervous system.)

Acupuncture brings about balance—relaxation—of the vital energy flow, thereby restoring equilibrium to the body organs. The question may be asked "How can acupuncture manipulation of body points make vital energy relax?" In answer we offer the following comparison: the manipulation of muscles makes them relax; it is, then, not illogical that manipulation of the vital energy at the body points makes the vital energy relax. We readily accept that manipulation of muscles relaxes them. It should not be too difficult to accept that manipulation of vital energy points can do the same for vital energy. In fact, since the musculature, nervous system and vital energy respond simultaneously to anything which happens to any one of them, massage of muscles simultaneously relaxes the vital energy and vice versa. When you press body points in a tense muscle area, you can easily feel the effect of the muscular tension on the points, and when the tension soreness in the muscles is reduced, tension soreness in the related body points will also be reduced.

We can expand the question of how puncture by a needle in a certain spot on the skin brings about relaxation (reestablishes vital energy balance) to read: how does applying pressure massage on a body point, or puncturing a body point, or heating a body point (moxa), produce relaxation? We might pursue the comparison as follows:

MANIPULATING THE MUSCLES by means of massage and pressure relaxes the muscles, both those directly involved and those in other parts of the body which relax in harmony with the muscles being massaged.

MANIPULATING THE BODY POINTS by means of massage, heat, or needles relaxes (rebalances) the vital energy flow and simultaneously the musculature, and particularly relaxes (rebalances) the specific organ system especially influenced by the points being manipulated.

If we thus compare the massage of muscles and its resultant relaxation with the manipulation of body points (massage, moxa, needles) and its resultant relaxation, the situations are really rather similar. We do not question the fact that massaging the muscles relaxes them, and we accept the physiological mechanics which must take place if manipulation of a muscle causes it, and many others throughout the musculature, to relax. If we can accept this for manipulating a muscle, we should be able to accept it for manipulating a body point without overly stretching the imagination.

151

HOW THE RESULTS OF RELAXATION VARY

The fact that acupuncture releases tension is generally known to therapists. The fact that this, primarily, may be the very reason acupuncture works does not seem to have been acknowledged.

The extraordinary effectiveness with which acupuncture relaxes is dramatically illustrated by its use to relieve muscle spasm. Applying needles to the proper points can bring immediate resolution of this condition. Muscle spasm is a convulsive, involuntary contraction—the relief of contraction is relaxation. Acupuncture needles accomplish this relaxation.

The argument may be proposed that acupuncture therapy sometimes sedates and sometimes stimulates, whereas relaxation is considered always to have a sedative effect. But, in actuality, relaxation is not necessarily a calming procedure (sedation), it can be stimulation. Remedial massage performed on body points by an acupuncture therapist is capable of either stimulating or toning down organ systems. Although the general layman's view of relaxation is that it calms down, what it really does is return the body to zero repose which is its balanced functioning condition, and this zero repose may mean either an increase or decrease in an organ system's activity, depending on whether it was previously hyper- or hypoactive.

For example, in the case of a person suffering from severe depression with concomitant tension/anxiety, several organ systems could be functioning below normal level due to the crippling tension. Depression is usually accompanied by anxiety which is inevitably accompanied by muscular tension. Relaxation of these tensions would serve to stimulate this person's organ systems, bringing them up to normal functioning level. We are not accustomed to thinking of relaxation as something which stimulates activity—but where function is below par due to the constricting effects of severe tension, the result of relaxation will naturally be stimulation. Depressed, anxiety/tension-ridden persons who succeed in achieving relaxation often experience a remarkable increase in vitality as a result.

152

Such a person's anxiety/depression had been forcing him into a "do nothing" lethargy, a lack of interest in his environment or in people. When relieved through relaxation, the person's systems begin functioning at normal energy levels—suddenly he wants to do things and is interested in what's going on around him. This is a toning up through relaxation, not sedating.

In cases of generalized fatigue, relaxation can also bring about overall stimulation of a person's entire system. The reason is that fatigue can be brought on by simple tension—because much greater than normal amounts of energy pour out of the body during tension (large quantities of energy are used up to maintain the muscular contractions of tension). By "simple tension" we mean the following: say a person has been setting up a new business—things are going well. So there's no pathological-type anxiety involved, just the normal stress of guiding a new venture. A certain tension accompanies this, and since the person is totally involved in his project, the concomitant tension is always with him. He never gives himself a chance to relax into any kind of repose, certainly not zero repose. Consequently, even during those moments when he's not actively working at, or thinking about, his project, larger than normal amounts of energy are still pouring out of his body because of the chronic tension. This uninterrupted, excessive emission of energy will soon make him feel fatigued. Even if he decides to take more time off from work to "rest", if his tension remains at all times close to peak effort level, that means his resting is going to be of limited benefit. Hard-driving, high-strung people often let go of only 5 or 10% of their tensions when "resting". If such a person should let go of at least 50%, preferably closer to 90% of his tensions, he'd put a stop to that tremendous waste of energy and the fatigue which results. When given a chance to recoup by relaxing down toward zero repose during its rest period, the body can return to full functioning at peak energy levels during its work period without unproductive tensions draining energy and interfering with performance. The body no longer suffers chronic fatigue due to continuous emission of

153

energy resulting from chronic simple tension since relaxation puts a stop to loss of this energy during non-effort-making (rest) periods. The result is recuperation, which does away with fatigue, which brings about a generally toned-up body able to work with new vitality when it returns to its tasks. Tension consumes energy; relaxation replenishes energy. Therefore, the end result of relaxation, in this case, has been stimulation, not sedation. (In this example, we speak only of the fatigue brought on by tension, not the type of fatigue which would result from pathological conditions such as long-standing bacterial infections, or the fatigue which is caused by plain old lack of sleep.)

AMONG THE MANY SPECIFIC BODY ACTIVITIES which tension suppresses and relaxation stimulates, sexual function is of major significance. We all know that with men, tension can make it difficult to have an erection or cause total impotence. In women, tension will inhibit sexual response, and can decrease the amount of menstrual flow to subnormal levels. A very large number of reproductive as well as other body functions can be impeded by tension and stimulated by relaxation.

Hysterical paralysis (non-organic paralysis due to psychological causes) can be relieved with acupuncture. Such paralysis results from extreme anxiety/tension conditions, and relaxation can stimulate activity in the paralysis-affected part of the body. It is relaxation that restores proper functioning (balance) wherever tension has distorted the balance.

To reiterate:

ACUPUNCTURE REESTABLISHES BALANCE.

RELAXATION REESTABLISHES BALANCE.

In a stomach that is tensed with anxiety, the secretions and digestive processes are not working in proper balance. In a stomach that is relaxed, juices are secreted in proper quantity and digestive processes proceed in a balanced manner (we refer, of course, to a normal person without

154

genetic, infectious, or tumor-caused malfunction).

Sometimes balance is reestablished in the human system by increasing function (stimulation), sometimes by decreasing it (sedation), sometimes by stimulation in some areas and sedation in others.

We are all familiar with how relaxation sedates hyperactivity; however, for the sake of completeness, we include the following examples:

A rather obvious case is insomnia. The insomniac knows that if he could only relax his mind, he would sleep—it's the hyperactivity in his brain that keeps him awake. Anxiety of some sort usually underlies the hyperactivity. Relaxation—calming—of the brain's activity brings sleep. Various relaxation techniques can help bring about the necessary calm, and acupuncture is particularly efficacious in doing so.

When heart palpitations are caused by nervous tension, any method of relaxation sedates the excess activity. Acupuncture, too, effectively calms the cardiac system to relieve hyperactivity such as palpitations.

HEAT TREATMENT OF VITAL ENERGY POINTS

The use of moxibustion in point treatment is of and by itself a persuasive argument in support of Relaxation Proof. Heat is a primary relaxant—utilizations familiar to us all are the heating pad and hot water bottle. (Naturally we refer to soothingly hot temperatures, not so hot as to cause discomfort or burns.) The most logical explanation for the benefits of moxibustion is the relaxant power of heat.

Catherine became very aware of this quality in heat when she was 17, a time during which she was subjected to enormous environmentally-caused stress. She discovered her own way of utilizing heat—she would take hot baths, sliding down into the water up to her chin, with the hot water faucet turned on slightly so that a continuous stream flowed into the tub. This increased the heat of the entire tub of water at a steady pace. When it was as hot as she could comfortably bear it, she turned off the faucet and soaked. Her whole body was a mass of tension which the

155

heat softened and relaxed—it also made her face perspire profusely and filled the entire bathroom with steam. Of course, numerous people have hit upon the super-hot bath method of relaxation, and other heat treatments such as steam baths can have similar effects. Nowadays, Cathy no longer uses the method, mainly because she's removed herself from the environment which inflicted the extreme stress, but also because she learned that long soakings in very hot water will dry out the skin.

What Cathy had been doing, in effect, with her super-hot baths was to heat-treat all her body points at one time. The musculature was, of course, simultaneously relaxed both directly by the heat and by the heat's effect on the points. Some may say a hot bath is simply general muscle relaxation, but with adequately hot water, the points must become treated. Just as general massage will affect the points and vital energy to some extent, since the masseur is bound to be manipulating body points when applying massage even though he may not know it, so a super-hot bath will inevitably heat-treat body points since they're all over the skin submerged in that hot water.

It's our opinion that heat applied to points will relax whether the individual knows about the existence of vital energy points or not. And heat knowingly applied to body points, by means of burning moxa, will also relax.

MASSAGE OF VITAL ENERGY POINTS

It's been said that point massage by an acupuncturist is different from Western massage because the purpose of point massage is to restore vital energy balance whereas Western massage simply manipulates muscles. We don't believe the purpose is different at all, we believe it's identical in all massage; namely, to relax the system, and restoration of vital energy balance takes place concurrently with relaxation. Regardless of what type of relaxation method you use, it will work toward restoring the vital energy balance. But acupressure massage is especially effective because the body points themselves are manipulated, and these points are where vital energy is accessible to us and can be directly influenced by us.

Since essentially the same therapeutic benefits can be achieved by simple massage of body points as are achieved by acupuncture, it would seem logical that the results are due to the same effect taking place in both instances. The effect which massage certainly achieves and acupuncture would logically also achieve is relaxation. Relaxed function is balanced function—and restoration of balance is the purpose of acupuncture.

There have been those among Western therapists who've recognized independently that plain massage also restores balance. During the 1920's, as an example, Mrs. E. Dicke, a German physical therapist, suffered a severe and painful illness that involved her right leg to the extent where amputation was recommended. She, however, succeeded in relieving and eventually curing her leg with the aid of a self-massage method which she devised. Mrs. Dicke, and later therapists using her method, concluded that this massage influenced the autonomic nervous system and by reflex action corrected imbalances in the functioning of internal systems. In our concept, the reflex action which restores the balance is relaxation.

It must be mentioned that we talk here of the kind of Western massage which is designed to soothe and relax—there are types of more forceful physical therapy manipulation which are rather severe and have purposes other than relaxation. However, it can easily be demonstrated that a normal, general massage has a soothing effect, and it's conceded that manual massage manipulation does bring about direct relaxation of voluntary muscles.

THE MOST POTENT ARGUMENT

The most potent argument verifying our statement that simple relaxation is the major reason why and how acupuncture works is the type of disorders for which it is used most effectively. These disorders lean heavily toward the kind which are caused by, or strongly influenced by, excessive and/or chronic tension/anxiety.

157

A second potent argument is the exceedingly large number of illnesses which are treatable by acupuncture— since so very many ailments can be treated by this one-and-the-same method, logic indicates there is a common denominator of cause, and of cure. We believe relaxation is the common denominator answer as to why and how acupuncture relieves and/or cures so vast a number of human ailments. And tension/stress/anxiety is the common denominator of cause.

Let us consider just the few following disorders which are among those most effectively treated by acupuncture: headaches, migraine, cramps, neuralgia, depression, anxiety, fatigue, hemorrhoids, nervous disorders, itching, sweating disorders, tics, certain types of paralysis, colitis, neuralgia, bed-wetting, constipation, impotence, insomnia. It's easy to see that tension plays a major role in these ailments and is often the direct, unequivocal cause.

Conversely, the diseases for which acupuncture treatment is least effective, or for which it provides only symptomatic relief, are of the following types: cancer, tuberculosis, infantile paralysis, mycotic infections. These are illnesses resulting from tissue degeneration or infectious organisms.

The entire picture presents a strong case for relaxation as the major reason why, and explanation of how, acupuncture works.

ACUPUNCTURE AND MENTAL HEALTH

The fact that acupuncture cures mental ailments of tension/anxiety origin also supports Relaxation Proof. The primary cure for such mental problems is relaxation; or, to put it another way, relaxation of the causative tension/anxiety is necessary in order for a cure to take place. Since acupuncture effects a cure, it must be bringing about relaxation.

Oriental medicine doesn't consider mind and body to be separate entities; "mental ailments" refers to conditions which do not, as yet, present overt physical symptoms. In acupuncture therapy, the patient is treated as a unit— there's no line of demarcation between mental and physical illness. No ailment is, in fact, isolated in the human system —any ailment, regardless how small, will have some repercussions on the entire system. Acupuncture, therefore, treats both the mental and physical aspects simultaneously.

The emotions—fear, frustration, anger, insecurity, hostility, aggravation—all affect the vital energy flow, all are reflected in tension and consequently sensitize the body points. Psychic tension is expressed in muscular tension. Passing emotions, even if violent, are harmless, since the human system is constructed to handle them without suffering permanent damage. But when emotions develop into severe cases of chronic anxiety/tension, organic ailments often result. Conversely, organic disturbances will cause mental anxiety, fear, and stress, and will affect the vital energy flow. Human ailments don't follow a fixed course in their development—they may start in the mind and develop symptoms in the body, or start in the body and affect the mind.

Those mental conditions curable by acupuncture have their source in anxiety/tension, as, for instance, maladjustment, neuroses, depression; whereas malignant brain tumors, infections, and such cannot be healed. Since the common denominator of cause for curable ailments is tension, the common denominator of cure is logically relaxation.

PULSE DIAGNOSIS AND RELAXATION PROOF

We talked about pulse diagnosis in the previous section titled "Acupuncture" and proposed that the reason it works may be that a certain organ isn't functioning in a healthy, rhythmically-balanced relationship with the blood (in receiving or supplying nutrients), and this reflects itself in the coursing of the blood, therefore also in the pulse. Here, in Relaxation Proof, we can take the matter one step further and propose tension as the reason the organ may not be functioning properly.

We drew the analogy between pulse diagnosis and hypertension. One of the factors which will raise blood pressure (cause hypertension) is mental anxiety/tension and the results of such emotional stress can easily be read on a machine (the sphygmomanometer). The coursing of blood through the veins is measurably altered by anxiety/tension. By the same token, tension interfering with the function of internal organs could reflect itself in how the blood flows, just as anxiety/tension reflects itself in blood pressure. Blood is a supply source of the human system and if an organ, such as the stomach, is thrown off balance by tension, the way it draws its requirements from blood would be affected by that distorted functioning. The dysfunction could then be read by sensory analysis of the blood flow at the pulses. Thus pulse diagnosis, too, may support our statement that tension is the common cause and relaxation the common denominator of cure for acupuncture-curable ailments.

LIVING HARMONIOUSLY

Also lending its support to Relaxation Proof is the fact that acupuncture theory states: an "unharmonious" life style will cause a condition which had been successfully cured to reappear in the same or in other forms. This is exactly the case with disorders resulting from tension/stress/anxiety. For example, if a stress/tension-caused condition such as headache is cured by acupuncture (or aspirin, for that matter) and the person continues to live in the same stress-laden environment which caused the headache, it will inevitably return after the aspirin or acupuncture has worn off. To take another example, if a child is successfully cured of bed-wetting and remains in the stress/tension-laden environment which caused this symptom, the child's problem will reappear either as renewed bed-wetting or in some other form. The same is indeed true of all conditions caused by tension/stress/anxiety and, regardless of what means is used to alleviate such a condition, it will return if the stress remains. Acupuncture therapy falls logically into the category of treatment for tension/stress-caused ailments, that treatment being relaxation of tension, since in order to accomplish a permanent cure, the stress/cause must be removed—or in acupuncture terminology, a "harmonious" life style must be assumed.

Chinese medicine states that in order to enjoy good health, one must have tranquility of mind, and eat a proper diet. The necessity of proper nutrients is recognized by all medical systems. The importance of relaxation or tranquility (relief from stress) is only now beginning to be recognized by Western medicine.

A certain amount of stress, however, is inevitable for most of us in life—indeed, experiencing some stress is completely normal to the process of living. Even the Chinese, who strived ardently for tranquility, recognized the inevitability of some stress, and their regimen for maintenance of health required a visit to one's acupuncturist once every six months (or once a year, if a person's health was unusually good). Thus any imbalance (tensions) which had built up could be corrected. When these imbalances did not yet present obvious symptoms, they were ascertained by pulse diagnosis.

Besides correcting particular conditions, acupuncture therapy has an overall effect on a person. Regardless of what ailment is being treated, any one of several general reactions may occur in the human system. Sometimes the reaction is one of lightness and buoyancy, a remarkable increase in energy, and a "feeling good" or "refreshed". Sometimes the general effect is a feeling of great repose, which may become a comfortable, contented drowsiness. In both cases, relaxation of tension can be the reason these responses are brought about. Also, patients who've received acupuncture treatments may find their sensory capabilities heightened—sounds and images will be sharper and brighter due to improved perception. Often thoughts become clearer, concentration better, the attention span longer, and general comprehension quicker and more complete. What one, common denominator factor brings about all these remarkable and highly desirable responses? Relaxation.

ACUPUNCTURE PAIN RELIEF AND RELAXATION PROOF

I've seen it written in several books to the effect that: "Massage will frequently relieve many types of pain, but

161

no one has given a clear-cut explanation of how this is accomplished". In other books, I've read words to the following effect: "Muscle tension causes pain, and that pain then causes you to tense your muscles even more which increases the pain". It is natural for a person to become more and more tense when in pain—we tense against the feeling of pain itself, and we tense with anxiety over a possible serious significance of the pain. The more the tension increases, the more the pain increases.

I've read the above two statements—"massage relieves pain" and "tension causes and increases pain" but have not seen anyone take the two and put them together: massage relaxes tension, thereby doing away with the pain which that tension caused. That is, of course, the answer: massage relieves pain because it relaxes the tension which had been responsible for causing or enhancing the pain. When pain is entirely due to tension, massage can remove it entirely.

Let us pursue the reasoning as follows:

1) Western-type massage (manipulation of muscles, which will inevitably include some vital energy points) relieves pain by relieving tension.

2) Acupressure massage (manipulation of vital energy points) relieves pain by relieving tension.

3) Puncturing the points (manipulation of vital energy points) relieves pain by relieving tension.

The effectiveness of acupuncture in relieving or removing pain has been widely heralded. How acupuncture accomplishes this has been considered a mystery. We believe it is accomplished primarily through relaxation of tension.

It's well known that if a person believes his stomach pain may be something serious, that pain often becomes excruciating. As soon as he learns it's only gas, his pain immediately subsides. Anxiety/tension increases pain for the same reason that pain occurs in the first place—to impress on you that something's not right, and unless you know the cause and know it's not serious, you'd better look into it. Pain is nature's alarm system which we must understand and appreciate.

The importance of relaxation—that is, relief of tension/

anxiety—in helping a patient minimize pain response is recognized by Western medicine. Many doctors, for instance, prescribe tranquilizers along with aspirin for a headache patient. When you hurt, it's difficult to relax. Besides the anxiety response, we also tense against the sensation of pain itself and tranquilizers help relieve these tensions. In addition to analgesics and sedatives, there are non-drug, mechanical means of relieving pain-influenced tensions; heat and massage, for instance, help a sore back because they help the muscles relax. And psychological approaches aid in calming down anxiety-tension, thereby reducing pain. As an example, reassurance helps the muscles relax—if a person who has broken a finger is assured it'll heal quickly and completely, his entire musculature relaxes (which means his anxiety/tension relaxes) and the pain decreases. Knowing a condition is transient and won't cause permanent damage eases tension and therefore pain. Putting a time limit on pain also eases it and often makes it bearable. Isabel had some minor dental work done recently and, since she didn't want novocain-stiff lips for several hours, she and the dentist agree to try without anesthetic. It went well, and afterwards Isabel commented "Some pain isn't difficult to bear if you know the cause and you know it's not going to last long". Under these conditions, tension/anxiety is at a minimum and therefore pain is at a minimum.

The fact that relaxation of tension/anxiety relieves pain fits neatly with Relaxation Proof of acupuncture's efficacy. Since piercing the body points with needles seems to greatly increase the degree of relaxation achieved, acupuncture becomes a more intensive application of what may be accomplished through use of an ordinary manipulative technique such as massage or heat.

However, now is a good time to reiterate that relaxation may not be the 100% answer to how and why acupuncture works. The next step after pain relief is use of acupuncture to achieve analgesia, and whether relaxation, by itself, could bring this about is a question which we have not, as yet, had the opportunity to research. But since analgesia has been accomplished solely by use of as simple a technique as autosuggestion, it would seem plausible that relaxation could also accomplish this. We cannot say it's a combination of autosuggestion and relaxation because acupuncture analgesia is effectively achieved on animals who are obviously not giving themselves anti-pain autosuggestions. It is possible that relaxation is the whole story. The situation may be similar to the fact that the brain does not produce images, but produces only the impulses for images and use of the musculature is necessary for an image to take place. Perhaps, in the same way, the nervous system produces only the impulse for pain and use of the musculature is necessary for the pain sensation to actually take place. Should this be the case, manipulation of vital energy by means of pulsating needles may be such a potent relaxant that the muscles do not contract, thus the sensation of pain does not occur.

In other words, what may happen is that the perpetual movement—pulsation or twirling—of needles piercing the points engenders such effective relaxation by means of the vital energy system that the necessary muscular contractions do not occur, and consequently pain sensation does not occur. But even if relaxation does prove to be the 100% answer, it is manipulation of vital energy, the controlling force, which is achieving this highly effective relaxation. Should it not prove to be the 100% answer, then some other aspect of the nature and behavior of vital energy will be involved.

IN CONCLUSION,

basically our main reasons for proposing that relaxation is the major factor in the why and how acupuncture works are as follows:

1. The type of ailments which acupuncture therapy treats most effectively are those caused by, or strongly influenced by, tension/anxiety.

2. The vast number of ailments treatable by acupunc-

ture supports the view that relaxation is a major factor in its efficacy since anxiety/tension is a contributory or causative factor in an enormous number of ailments, and these all have relaxation as a common means of relief or cure.

3. The fact that heat (which relaxes) and massage (which relaxes) applied to the body points can accomplish, to a great extent, the same results as piercing the points with needles seems to confirm that relaxation is a major factor in acupuncture therapy.

4. The fact that applying pressure precisely on a body point by using a narrow, round-tipped rod instead of using a comparatively broad fingertip will increase the relaxation effectiveness tends to support Relaxation Proof in acupuncture since it's only a very short step from use of a slender rounded tip to a sharp tip which will pierce the body point. It is logical that increased intensification of action at the point by use of a sharp tip which pierces will further increase the relaxation effectiveness.

5. In order for an organ or any element of the human system to function in a balanced manner, it must be relaxed. Any tension will inevitably bring about imbalance, however slight the tension and corresponding imbalance may be. Acupuncture restores balance to the human system, both to the entire system and any part thereof. In order to restore balance, any existing tension must be relaxed; therefore, acupuncture must bring about relaxation.

WE HAVE ONE FINAL OBSERVATION

to make regarding acupuncture, an observation dealing with an aspect of this medical art which we haven't, as yet, talked about; namely, the theory that acupuncture restores harmony between the human being and the cosmos. Acupuncture considers a person, mind and body, to be an indivisible Whole, but that Whole is not an entity existing of and by itself in aloof isolation. On the contrary, that Whole, which is the human being, is an integral part of the greater Whole, which is the cosmos. And to function at his best, the human being should function in harmony with the cosmos.

The great cosmic Whole (the universe) is permeated with a fundamental force which we shall call the "basic-energy" (hyphenated because it's more accurately one word than two). All things, animate and inanimate, are permeated with their own specific manifestations of this basic-energy. Human vital energy is one such manifestation.

But all human V-energy is not the same—each person has his own individual version of it. Thus, each human's vital energy is part of the intricate pattern of general human vital energy—which is part of the even more complex cosmic basic-energy.

Acupuncture therapy, it is said, puts the patient in harmony with the cosmos. It establishes balance not only within an individual's human system but also between that human and the universe of which he is a part. How can acupuncture accomplish such a wondrous feat, one which is impressive to the point of being quite overwhelming? It's easy. Relaxation puts you in harmony with the cosmos.

When your human system is quite relaxed, you naturally function at your own rhythm in accordance with the great cosmic pattern of basic-energy, the all-pervasive and all-creative universal force. Your vital energy was created as part of the cosmic pattern; the combined forces of your vital energy and the great cosmic energy determine your natural rhythm. When you do not upset your natural rhythm but function in harmony with it, you're functioning in harmony with the cosmic environment.

Even as you go about contracting certain areas of your musculature in order to perform the actions necessary and pertinent to the process of living (ambulation, food gathering, self cleansing, reproduction, construction of shelter, intellectual and creative activity, etc.) you are still functioning at your natural rhythm (harmoniously) as long as you function from a base of relaxation and only those muscular contractions necessary to the action are em-

166

ployed. What puts you out of harmony are the chronic/
excessive/unnecessary tensions which interfere with the
normal contractions used in each action. It is the relaxation of these tensions that restores your natural biorhythm
and concurrently your harmony within yourself and with
the cosmos. In addition, since tension consumes energy
and relaxation replenishes energy, your full resources become available for productive use, which means total
living.

Any relaxation method, such as yoga or prayer-type
meditation, will help put you in harmony with the cosmos.
If you just sit down comfortably and consciously let your
muscles go (relax the excessive/unnecessary/chronic tensions), you are progressing toward harmony with the cosmos. The difference is mainly in efficacy of the various
methods and, of them all, vital energy manipulation is far
and away the most powerful relaxant. You cannot use
acupuncture yourself, but in acupressure, you literally have
at your fingertips a safe, easy means of influencing your
own vital energy.

When simple relaxation can give you the benefits of
cosmic harmony, renewed energy, living in accord with
your natural biorhythm, and functioning at your optimum
performance level for the fullest, richest participation in
life, it is certainly worth pursuing. Especially since all you
need to gain relaxation is a little time and some knowledge
of acupressure.